Each Day I Like It Better

D1474336

Each Day I Like It Better

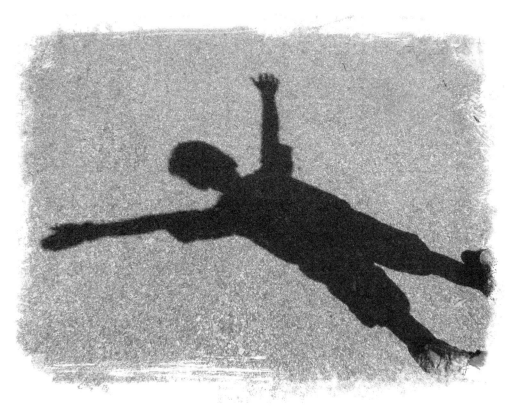

AUTISM, ECT, AND THE
TREATMENT OF OUR MOST
IMPAIRED CHILDREN

AMY S. F. LUTZ

VANDERBILT UNIVERSITY PRESS

Nashville

Published 2014 by Vanderbilt University Press
Nashville, Tennessee 37235

This book is printed on acid-free paper.
Manufactured in the United States of America

Frontispiece photograph by Amy Lutz
Text design by Rich Hendel
Composition by Vanderbilt University Press

Library of Congress Cataloging-in-Publication Data on file
LC control number 2013034804
LC classification number RJ506.A9L88 2013
Dewey class number 618.92'85882—dc23

ISBN 978-0-8265-1975-7 (hardcover)
ISBN 978-0-8265-1976-4 (paperback)
ISBN 978-0-8265-1977-1 (ebook)

For Jonah,

Matthew, Paul,

Gary, David, Sam,

John, and Alex

Contents

Foreword   xi
by Charles Kellner, MD, and Dirk Dhossche, MD

1   JONAH, 2009
The Debate on Cognitive Side Effects   1

2   MATTHEW   22

3   JONAH, JANUARY–MARCH 2010
The Efficacy Studies   31

4   PAUL   44

5   JONAH, MARCH 2010
ECT Begins   52

6   GARY AND DAVID   67

7   JONAH, MARCH–APRIL 2010
One Step Forward, Two Steps Back   76

8   SAM   99

9   JONAH, APRIL 2010
Maintenance Begins   106

10   ALEX   120

11   JONAH, AUGUST–SEPTEMBER 2010
How Does ECT Work?   139

12   JOHN   150

13   THE ECT CONTROVERSY   160

Epilogue, January 26, 2011: The FDA Hearing   175

Afterword, May 16, 2013   185

Acknowledgments   189

Notes   191

Index   197

If love were the cure,

I would have been healed

a long time ago.

— Martha Manning,
  *Undercurrents: A Life
  Beneath the Surface*

Foreword

BY CHARLES KELLNER, MD, & DIRK DHOSSCHE, MD

"You don't still use ECT, and surely not in children, do you?" is the first question often blurted out by parents, medical professionals, and lay people when they hear that electroconvulsive therapy (ECT) is recommended as a potential treatment for a child or adolescent. The question is fraught with the prejudice and views promulgated by the anti-psychiatric movement since the 1970s and epitomized in the movie *One Flew Over the Cuckoo's Nest.* It is also the first issue that Amy Lutz grapples with when finding out that ECT may benefit her nine-year-old son, Jonah, by relieving his unrelenting self-injury and aggressive rages.

Yet ECT comes out as the dark horse in *Each Day I Like It Better: Autism, ECT, and the Treatment of Our Most Impaired Children.* A courageous mother chronicles the effects of ECT in her child and several other children and adolescents with developmental delay. She believes that the benefits of ECT refute what she calls the "*Cuckoo's Nest* culture." We agree.

This book gives a first-hand account of the daily struggles of a family with the profoundly disruptive, out-of-control behaviors that some children with autism exhibit. It chronicles the journey that this family undertakes when ECT is recommended, and pursued, with considerable effort and persistence, in a collaboration between parents and physicians.

Amy and Andy Lutz first came to Mount Sinai Hospital in New York in 2009 for an ECT consultation, desperate for help for Jonah, who had been in an escalating manic state for two months. Jonah was too ill to be present at the consultation. ECT proved to be successful and life-changing in curbing the behaviors that otherwise would have required the child's placement in a residential treatment setting away from the family.

ECT is not portrayed as a cure for autism. Amy Lutz tells about her hopes, fantasies, doubts, anxieties, desperation, and ultimately, relief when she sees the improvement in her son brought about by ECT and then maintenance ECT. The book is filled with heartfelt details, at times amusing, at times wrenching, but always informative for other parents who may face similar situations and difficulties when they explore ECT as a treatment option for their children.

As clinical scientists, we believe that the finding that reducing intractable repetitive acts of self-injury and aggressive rage in children with autism spectrum disorders may be a new indication for ECT has substantial scientific importance. The recommendation to use ECT for Jonah and the other children portrayed in this book was deliberate, not haphazard, based on theory and previous experience with ECT use in catatonia and mood disorders, both accepted clinical indications for ECT.

As academic ECT practitioners, we are impressed with the amount and scope of research on ECT and its history collected here but would also like to offer readers a basic understanding of the treatment so that they may more fully appreciate the clinical stories in this book.

ECT remains a controversial treatment for neurotypical adults, let alone for children with autism; however, it should not be, for either group. ECT is a mainstream treatment in modern psychiatry, and yet misperceptions about how it is done and what it is prescribed for continue, fueled largely by sensational media misrepresentations. Only abortion tops ECT as a controversial medical procedure.

ECT was invented in 1938, at a time when modern anesthesia techniques had not yet been developed. This early form of ECT, now referred to as "unmodified ECT," was unfortunately done without any anesthesia or muscle relaxation. The frightening scene in *One Flew Over the Cuckoo's Nest*, in which Jack Nicholson's charcter is forced to undergo unmodified ECT, has remained the dominant image of ECT. Modern ECT bears no resemblance to the outmoded technique depicted in the movie.

ECT in contemporary psychiatric medicine is used to treat a limited number of severe psychiatric illnesses, usually mood or psychotic disorders in adults. While not really a treatment of "last resort," it is usually recommended only after antidepressant and antipsychotic medications have been ineffective in relieving acute symptoms of depression or psychosis. For a small number of urgently ill patients, ECT is recommended as an initial treatment because it is so reliably effective and works quickly. For very suicidal patients or those whose weight loss from depression threatens their health, ECT can be lifesaving.

Modern ECT is administered as a series of treatments under full general anesthesia and muscle relaxation. When used to treat severe depression (by far the most common indication), a course of ECT, usually six to twelve treatments, is continued until the depressive symptoms have resolved. Because depression is an episodic, relapsing illness, ECT is typically stopped when the episode of depression is fully treated. Most patients are then continued on antidepressant and other psychotropic medications to stabilize their moods and to prevent subsequent episodes of depression. For patients with a history of frequent episodes of depression that are not prevented by medications, a form of intermittent ECT, called "maintenance ECT," can be considered. This is usually done in an outpatient setting at a frequency ranging from every two to eight weeks.

The efficacy, safety, and side effects of ECT in children and adolescents are similar to those in adults. Modern clinical reviews on the use of ECT in children and adolescents report excellent improvement rates for depression, schizophrenia, mania, and catatonia. Prospective studies of ECT for psychotropic-refractory depression in adolescents also document significant clinical improvement. It is important to recognize that severe depression, mania, and schizophrenia typically present in adolescence rather than early childhood, thus reducing the likelihood of need for ECT in younger children for such indications. In adolescents, current studies support the use of ECT for the same indications as in adults and report equal clinical efficacy.

ECT is a remarkably safe procedure in adults, and there is no reason to believe that ECT is any less safe in children. In fact, because much of the medical morbidity and most of the (very rare) mortality of ECT is from cardiac events in elderly patients with severe cardiac disease, ECT is likely much safer in children. It is known that children have lower seizure thresholds than older patients and tend to have longer ECT seizures. For these reasons, the electrical stimulus dose used in pediatric ECT is considerably lower than that of adults. ECT practitioners who treat children are aware of the possibility of prolonged seizures, and are ready to end a seizure over 180 seconds in duration. This is typically done by administering additional anesthetic or intravenous benzodiazepine. The concern that the "developing brain" is vulnerable to ECT-induced damage is not supported by any credible evidence; on the other hand, there is reason to suspect that prolonged periods of severe depression or catatonia may be harmful to the brain. Recent evidence suggests that ECT, like other antidepressant treatments, may have neuroprotective and neurotropic effects.

A considerable body of basic and clinical science data (over ten thousand citations on PubMed) documents the many profound neurobiological effects ECT has on brain function. We know that monoamine neurotransmitter systems are enhanced, similar to the way antidepressant medications are believed to work. For example, hypothalamic-pituitary-adrenal (HPA) axis dysfunction, a biochemical abnormality implicated in certain disorders, is corrected by a course of ECT. Paradoxically, ECT is a potently anticonvulsant treatment: ECT recruits inhibitory brain mechanisms that turn off seizures. This is demonstrated by the fact that ECT-induced seizures become shorter and harder to elicit later in a course of treatment. The neurotropic effects of ECT are well described in animal experiments that show increased neurogenesis in the dentate gyrus of the rat hippocampus, and in human studies that show increased brain-derived neurotrophic factor (BDNF) release. Yet, despite this wealth of knowledge, the specific brain change or changes that cause the antidepressant, antipsychotic, and anticatatonic effects of ECT are not fully understood. In large part this is because the underlying causes of the psychiatric illnesses for which ECT is effective are not at all well understood. The full explanation of the mechanism of action of ECT will likely need to await the understanding of the etiology of psychiatric illness. Fortunately, the pace of neuroscience discovery is accelerating, aided greatly by advances in neuroimaging and genetics, so there is reason to hope that explanations will be forthcoming. Of course, such explanations will be comforting to both patients and practitioners. In the meantime, however, we do not feel that our incomplete knowledge base about the mechanism of action should be a credible reason to deny patients a proven, safe, and effective medical treatment.

No discussion of ECT is complete without mention of the cognitive effects of the treatment, about which reams have been written and about which controversy continues to swirl. In fact, like the broader controversy that surrounds ECT itself, the controversy around cognition is overblown, fueled by misinformation and exaggeration. Contemporary ECT causes far less memory loss than ECT of the past. For most patients, this side effect is a reasonable trade-off for relief from a debilitating illness. ECT interferes with the encoding of new memories for the few weeks of the treatment course; sometimes it erases some memory for the weeks or, more rarely, the months preceding the treatments. Some of those memories come back; some do not. Memory functioning returns to normal within weeks after ECT for the vast majority of patients. We believe an appropriate medical analogy is the side effects of chemotherapy: hair loss and "chemo brain" are unpleasant side effects, but most patients would choose the potentially life-saving therapy. Maintenance ECT is given at such extended intervals that memory loss is rarely a problem.

There are, as yet, no controlled trials of ECT in autism. Several recent reports document the efficacy of ECT in autistic adolescents with catatonia, and ECT is included in standard treatment algorithms for autistic catatonia when benzodiazepines prove insufficient or patient morbidity is severe. Indeed, autistic catatonia is of high clinical relevance in child psychiatry, given that catatonia may be seen in up to one out of six autistic patients (17 percent) and may cause significant clinical impairment. ECT-responsive malignant catatonia—a severe, life-threatening form of the illness—has also been reported in patients with autism. None of the reports indicate cognitive or functional decline after ECT.

We hope that the clinical evidence for the use of ECT to treat autistic catatonia and autistic self-injury and aggression will lead to support for clinical trials that will definitively establish the proper role of ECT in the treatment of these children. The inspiring collaborations between the families and their physicians described in this book have already advanced the field of autism treatment. We thank Amy Lutz and these families for having the courage and determination to share their stories.

CHAPTER 1

Jonah, 2009

THE DEBATE ON COGNITIVE SIDE EFFECTS

NOVEMBER 20, 2009

Crisis, I've discovered, is a relative term.

When the care manager who coordinates the services my autistic ten-year-old son, Jonah, gets from the State of Pennsylvania asks me if I'm in crisis, I'm not sure how to answer.

Is it a crisis if your son has just attacked your tiny Thai au pair, even if he hits you or his father or his teacher or his aides every day? What if you're afraid that your son's aggression toward the au pair represents an expansion of his range of potential targets, so that now you won't only have to anticipate Jonah coming after the adults in charge, but also strangers in Costco, or neighbors over for dinner? What if this isn't an isolated incident, because Jonah also recently hit one of his sisters and your greatest fear of all is that, instead of ignoring the seven other young children who live in your house—kids who obviously irritate Jonah with their shrieking, their intrusions, their stubborn fearlessness—he may start unleashing his rage against his siblings and his cousins? Is that crisis?

Apparently, at four-thirty on a Friday afternoon, insurance company managers have no patience for the nuances of crisis. Mine gives me the number of a psychiatric facility where I can take Jonah for an emergency evaluation.

I hang up the phone and call the hospital. A receptionist tells me that I should take Jonah to the local emergency room because "we don't really treat autistic kids here."

I call the insurance company back, wondering if anyone will even answer, since it's now past five. My manager is still there. He puts me on hold while, I suppose, he calls the facility and berates them into agreeing to do the assessment.

"I'm not taking Jonah someplace that doesn't work with autistic kids," I say.

I can tell he's getting impatient with me: first, I call him late on a Friday afternoon in a panic over Jonah's escalating violence and my fear that he may need another hospitalization to adjust his medications, then I reject the only offer he's able to scrape together on such short notice. He says that if I can't wait until Monday I have no other options.

"I can wait," I say. What would clearly be a crisis for virtually everyone I know is just a more intense level of the kind of behaviors we've been struggling with since Jonah was a toddler. "My husband will be home soon. We can manage."

Yes, we manage. We're very fortunate to have a lot of support. My sister, Keri, her husband, Matty, and their young kids, Declan (5), Ronan (3½), and Molly (1½), live with us. Matty has, on many occasions, stepped in front of a raging Jonah to spare me the brunt of an attack. We also have two childcare helpers who free me up to work one-on-one with Jonah, as well as a veritable stable of aides who free me up to spend time with my four other children: Erika (8), Hilary (6), and twins Aaron and Gretchen (3½). But I don't always feel so lucky. Managing Jonah's behavior occupies us 24/7. It dictates the places we can and can't go, the things we can and can't do, and often necessitates that we split up, with one of us—usually my husband, Andy—taking Jonah to the wholesale clubs he loves so much, with their walk-in freezers, their mysteriously appealing stacks of tires, and their enormous sheet cakes. Meanwhile I take my four younger kids to their swimming lessons, to the movies, to family functions Jonah has no patience for.

We've tried everything to control Jonah's behaviors. At first, we were drawn to the alternative routes popular in the autistic community: we kept Jonah on a gluten- and casein-free diet for four years, and experimented with probiotics, B12 injections, auditory integration training, topical chelation, and hyperbaric oxygen therapy. When these didn't help, we turned to psychiatry. Over the past six years, Jonah has been prescribed anticonvulsants that made him fat; stimulants that made him more agitated; antidepressants that made him manic; antihypertensives that did nothing at all; and anti-psychotics that helped a little, but never enough, and made him even heavier. Now he takes lithium and Abilify, a cocktail created for him at the Kennedy Krieger Institute in Baltimore, where Jonah spent most of 2008 as a patient on the Neurobehavioral Unit (NBU). The NBU takes developmentally delayed kids with the very worst behaviors—teens so aggressive it takes seven armor-clad therapists to manage their outbursts, and children so self-injurious they wear helmets and padding so they don't smash their heads against the walls or bite chunks out of their own arms. When Jonah was discharged from the NBU, with a diagnosis of rapid-cycling bipolar disorder with catatonic features to tack onto the autism diagnosis he'd been given at age two, he was fairly stable. Now, almost a year later, that's no longer the case. In the past several weeks we've seen a ferocity in his tantrums we haven't seen since before he was admitted to the NBU. Last month, while Jonah was riding in the car, he flew into a rage, whacking his head against the window and trying to kick, punch, and bite both Andy and the aide who was with them. Desperate to keep Jonah from attacking his grandfather, who was driving, Andy tried to restrain him. He ended up snapping Jonah's arm. I will never forget running into the emergency room and finding my typically hyperactive son lying immobile on a gurney, asking surreally for a Band-Aid, while Andy sobbed over and over, "I'm sorry, I'm so sorry." Neither of us could say what I know we both were thinking: *How much longer can we do this?*

I hang up the phone after my conversation with the care manager, feeling completely alone although right now there are fourteen other people in my house. Andy is still at work. Jonah is, for the time being, working quietly with his aide. The other kids are watching a movie in the basement, two floors beneath my feet. Keri and Matty are getting ready to go out with guests visiting from New York, a high school friend and her husband. I had seen them briefly in the kitchen, pretending they didn't hear Jonah's intermittent screams, notice his chapped and swollen hands, or hear that he had attacked the au pair. And I want to go down there and tell them—as I want to explain to everyone who's witnessed one of Jonah's violent outbursts—that this isn't really Jonah, that these uncontrollable tantrums are part of his disorder, that at his core Jonah is a sweet, affectionate, funny kid who loves water parks and roller coasters and deliberately misquoting lines from his favorite videos. I want to tell them that these fits are aberrations, but I just don't know if I believe that anymore. When something is as persistent as this rage has been; when it recurs again and again, despite the drugs and the behavior plans; when even the brightest minds in psychiatry and behavior can only control it for brief periods—well, when do you declare that something to be essential, not just an aberration? All this time, I think, burying my head in my hands. I really believed, all this time, we would beat this thing.

The phone rings on the desk next to my ear, right where I dropped it. It's Dr. Lee Wachtel, Jonah's psychiatrist at Kennedy Krieger. We haven't seen Dr. Wachtel in almost a year, but she was the first person I called after I came home and found out about Jonah's attack on Oat, our au pair. Not only does Dr. Wachtel know Jonah's history, but I can't think of anyone more experienced with the gamut of pharmacological and behavioral interventions used to treat this population. She stabilized Jonah once. Maybe, I had thought as I left what I'm sure was a frantic, semi-coherent message on her voicemail, she could help me stabilize him again.

Dr. Wachtel was calling from home. "I just got your message," she says. "I was going to wait until Monday to call you back, but you sounded so upset I thought I'd better check in."

It's a relief just to hear her voice. I tell her everything that's been going on, from Andy breaking Jonah's arm, to Jonah hitting Hilary in the car, to his aggression toward the au pair. I tell her that the medications are no longer working and I'm scared to experiment at home. I know the waiting list for the NBU is long, at times a year or more, but maybe she knows of another respected ward where Jonah's medications could be safely adjusted?

Dr. Wachtel tells me about Shepherd Pratt, another facility in Maryland I had researched online before our admission to Kennedy Krieger. She agrees that it sounds like Jonah may need a second hospitalization. We talk about some of the other drugs that might be helpful, including riluzole, which we had tried at the end of Jonah's stay on the NBU, but discontinued because it didn't seem to help. Dr. Wachtel suspected the riluzole might not have worked because it was supposed to be taken on an empty stomach; at that time Jonah took all his medicine in a peanut butter sandwich because he couldn't swallow pills. Riluzole significantly helped another patient who was on the unit while Jonah was there, a teenager who had previously been so violent that whenever he was moved around the NBU one of his many aides would holler, "Mark's in the North Tower/South Tower/ Common Room!" so everyone knew to get out of the way. Riluzole was added to Mark's regimen following his acute course of ECT, Dr. Wachtel explains, and now he's getting ready to be discharged to a group home.

While Jonah was on the NBU, I knew that electroconvulsive therapy (ECT) was used on some of the more intractable patients, but Dr. Wachtel had never suggested we consider it because Jonah initially responded so well to the new medications. Now, however, I wonder aloud: "Did you ever think ECT might help Jonah?"

Dr. Wachtel pauses. And then she talks for a long time, the hope evident in her voice. The short answer is yes, she thinks Jonah could benefit from ECT. She's used it on eleven kids with extreme behaviors who failed to respond after numerous medication trials, and all eleven showed substantial improvement. As I know, the NBU has a long waiting list, but Dr. Wachtel has colleagues in other hospitals who have also been extremely successful using ECT to treat kids like Jonah—doctors at facilities in Jackson, Mississippi; Ann Arbor, Michigan; and the closest to me, New York, who boast an impressive 80 percent remission rate.

Because of my casual exposure to ECT on the NBU, I know that it no longer looks anything like the torture depicted in *One Flew Over the Cuckoo's Nest*—and that it didn't even look like that in 1962 when Ken Kesey wrote the book upon which the movie was based. Since the late 1950s, ECT has been performed under general anesthesia, with muscle relaxants to prevent patients from thrashing. Still, Kesey's anachronistic images continue to define the procedure for most laypeople and even for many doctors. Despite a mountain of scientific evidence documenting the safety and efficacy of ECT—studies Dr. Wachtel promises to send me—vocal anti-ECT lobbies, including the Church of Scientology, have compared treatment of patients with ECT to torture, crimes against humanity, and the practices of Nazi doctors during the Holocaust.

I promise to read the studies and to pursue additional research on my own—and I will. But what I don't tell Dr. Wachtel is that my decision has already been made. More accurately, there is no decision to make: a decision requires multiple choices, and it's obvious to me that we have run out of options. I can't help thinking about the months Jonah was at Kennedy Krieger and how many times well-meaning friends patted me on the shoulder and sympathetically murmured, *That must have been such a difficult decision.* They seemed so surprised when I corrected them that after a while I just stopped saying that it was, in fact, one of the easiest decisions we ever made. Jonah's school had expelled him, his psychiatrist was confounded by him. After all our failed interventions, taking him anywhere other than Kennedy Krieger, widely respected as one of the best treatment centers in the world for kids with dangerous behaviors, would have felt like giving up.

And now, what are our choices? Another hospitalization? Different combinations of the same kinds of hardcore psychotropics we've been pumping into Jonah since he was five years old? Honestly, it's hard to imagine anything about ECT could scare me as much as antipsychotics. This most common family of medications used to treat aggression in autistic children has a truly alarming side-effect profile: acute dystonia (severe muscular cramping), akathisia (a frantic and reportedly unbearable restlessness usually described as feeling like "ants in your pants"), tardive dyskinesia (a transient or permanent syndrome of abnormal, involuntary movements), glaucoma, and neuroleptic malignant syndrome (a potentially fatal reaction to antipsychotics that presents with fever, stiffness, delirium, and autonomic system instability). In her book *We've Got Issues: Children and Parents in the Age of Medication*, Judith Warner reports that over two hundred children died between 2000 and 2006 due to complications from antipsychotic use, and she takes pains to point out that, because reporting these reactions to the FDA is not mandated by law, the number is likely much higher.

This list doesn't even include the most ubiquitous side effect—weight gain—which is so common it's taken for granted, although it obviously predisposes patients to significant health problems, such as diabetes and heart disease. A 2006 study reported that these chronic conditions contribute to a significantly abbreviated life span for patients treated in public mental facilities—an average *twenty-five years* shorter than that of the general population. When Jonah was admitted to Kennedy Krieger, the first thing Dr. Wachtel did was wean him off the Risperdal that, although it failed to improve his behavior, did earn him a new diagnosis—obesity—to add to his growing list of labels. By the time he was discharged, Jonah had dropped twenty-four pounds—almost a quarter of his initial body weight.

After Dr. Wachtel offers to send me the contact information of parents whose children have been treated with ECT, I let her go back to her own kids, whom I hear clamoring for her attention in the background. *Eleven out of eleven*, I think, as I hang up. It's hard to argue with those numbers.

When Jonah was first diagnosed, I spent a lot of time looking for what I referred to as "Jonah's miracle." Since the first book we read about autism was Karyn Seroussi's account of how her son was virtually cured by a gluten- and casein-free diet, (*Unraveling the Mystery of Autism and Pervasive Developmental Disorder*, Simon & Schuster, 2000). Andy and I hoped that diet would be Jonah's miracle as well. After four years of soy pretzels and rice pasta, we realized the diet wasn't helping. Other candidates for Jonah's miracle included the melatonin we started giving him when he was four that caused a substantial improvement in his behavior, but only for a few months; the forty hyperbaric oxygen treatments that would have definitely bought us a miracle, if one could be purchased with enough time or money; even the lithium, which we had erroneously imagined as the missing puzzle piece that would meet the jagged edges of Jonah's bipolar disorder and create a complete and harmonious design suitable for framing.

We don't talk much about miracles anymore. Now that Jonah's almost eleven, it's clear he won't be the handsome but socially awkward math geek who can't be pried away from his computer by the hottest coeds M.I.T. has to offer, as Andy and I used to joke. Now when I dwell upon the future, my thoughts evolve into a prayer of sorts about the life I *don't* want for Jonah: a locked ward, heavy sedation, restraints. Jonah is likely to be big and strong like his father, who is 6'1" and weighs over 220 pounds. Even if he only has violent tantrums once a week or even once a month—a huge reduction from his current, medicated level of aggression—they will still preclude him from working, participating in the community, and staying with us or transitioning to a group home.

On February 6, 2009, Kent State Professor Trudy Steuernagel died following a brutal beating at the hands of her nineteen-year-old autistic son, Sky Walker. It chilled me to read the parts of this heart-breaking story that echoed our struggles with Jonah: how smart Trudy always said Sky was, when he was in a good mood; the obsessions with food that often fueled Sky's tantrums; Trudy's persistent hope, despite the medicine cabinet filled with useless prescriptions, that doctors would find the right cocktail of drugs that would stabilize Sky's behavior. Then, the ominous warning that echoed what I had heard before—how Sky's violence escalated during puberty, a common pattern in autistic boys. Jonah, two months shy of his eleventh birthday, is just starting to go through adolescence; when his arm was in a cast from shoulder to thumb, we tried to stretch his daily showers to once every two or three days and discovered that it was time for him to start using deodorant. There isn't a day that goes by now that I don't think, *we haven't got much time*.

So no, we don't talk about miracles anymore. But, regardless of whether we are objectively, officially, "in crisis," it's clear we need one, more than ever. Sitting in my office, the phone lying belly-up on the desk in front of me, I recognize the excitement humming along my nerves—it's the same giddy hope I felt when my school district agreed to pay over $60,000 a year to send Jonah to the Nexus School, a lovely little private school for autistic children that kicked him out less than a week after he transferred there; that I felt again when Kennedy Krieger called after four months of home-schooling to say that a bed had finally opened up for Jonah. It was that feeling that never really goes away, whether or not you articulate it: *Maybe this could be Jonah's miracle*.

DECEMBER 7, 2009

As we drive up to Mount Sinai Hospital in Manhattan to discuss whether Jonah might be a good candidate for ECT with Dr. Charles Kellner, I can't help thinking about another car ride Andy and I took about eight years ago. Like this one, that trip felt momentous. We knew as the day approached that it would be one we would always remember, and my feelings that morning were similar: anxious, yet hopeful. As I do today, I had a list of questions folded in my bag because we were finally meeting with someone who had Answers, and I didn't trust myself to remember everything we needed to ask. But that time I only had about half an hour to fidget in the car because, instead of driving the hundred miles to New York City, we were going to the Children's Hospital of Philadelphia (CHOP) to hear the results of the battery of tests the developmental pediatrician had given Jonah the week before.

It wasn't as if we didn't already know. Six months before, at Jonah's two-year-old check-up, our pediatrician had expressed concern that Jonah wasn't talking. We weren't worried about it yet as it was clear—and I say this without irony, without sarcasm—Jonah was brilliant. By the time he was eighteen months old, he was crawling around the pool table, lining all the balls up in order. And he couldn't have been more charming, friendly, or affectionate. I know I'm not misremembering because it wasn't just my opinion. Once we were out with our friends Chris and Katrina, whose son is one month younger than Jonah, and Chris remarked, "With Andrew's looks and Jonah's personality, they're going to get all the girls." I remember thinking, *How about with JONAH's looks and Jonah's personality, etc.*, because my son was perfect: beautiful, smart, happy, charismatic.

Maybe there were early signs, but we didn't see them. In 2000, autism hadn't yet captured the public consciousness as it would by the middle of the decade. The general perception of autism was the one embodied by Dustin Hoffman in *Rain Man*: disengaged, extremely sensitive to touch, savant in some impressive manner. Many of the childcare bibles I had on my shelf, like *What to Expect the First Year*, included developmental checklists at the end of every chapter, but none of them mentioned the first indicators of a spectrum disorder that few parents—especially first-timers like us—would know to look for: pointing with a clear, index-finger point; responding to name; following simple, one-step directions. When Jonah was about fifteen months old, those same friends came over and when it was time to leave, Chris told Andrew to get his shoes. Neither of the boys was talking at all; they had just recently begun walking, but Andrew toddled off to retrieve his shoes. I remember wondering, *Wow, when will Jonah be able to do that?* So there might have been other signs I would recognize now. Certainly my pediatrician saw something that caused him to recommend at that two-year check-up that we begin the evaluation process.

That night when Andy got home from work, I told him about our upcoming appointment with a hearing specialist. "The doctor said that all developmental screenings start with a hearing test," I said. "Jonah might not be talking because he's deaf!"

Andy shook his head. He walked into the family room where Jonah was watching *The Best of Kermit*, his favorite video, and turned off the sound. Jonah grabbed Andy's hand, pushing it toward the volume knob on the receiver, which sat on top of the TV. "He's not deaf," Andy said. I wouldn't have been so relieved if I had understood we had just witnessed a classic early sign of autism: using another person as a tool. A typical toddler would have pointed at the receiver, a gesture that indicates joint attention. This milestone of early development reflects the toddler's recognition that he and his parent are both looking at the same object, as well as his desire that his parent share his interest in that object. For Jonah, at that moment, Andy was nothing more than a giant knob-turning device.

The next step in the process was an assessment by a team from our county's Early Intervention program. That report was similarly unenlightening since the evaluators—a speech therapist, a psychologist, and a teacher—were prohibited from even suggesting a diagnosis, but over the next few months, the gaps between Jonah and his peers became more and more apparent. By the time our appointment with the developmental pediatrician at CHOP rolled around in August, when Jonah was past two-and-a-half, he had been working with an Early Intervention therapist and a private speech pathologist for months. He didn't speak at all, but after countless repetitions, he had mastered one sign: *more*. Formed by touching the fingertips of both hands together, Jonah got a lot of mileage out of that sign and used it to ask for anything, whether he'd already had some or not. I remember watching the technician at CHOP administer the tests through a one-way mirror and thinking, *Just let her see him sign 'more.'* It was like a mantra in my head—*Sign 'more,' Jonah, please let her see you sign 'more'*—until that moment when my son, so small then, standing with his head craned back to watch the technician and her bright bottle of bubble liquid, finally tapped his fingertips together: more bubbles. I'm not sure why it was so important to me, but I remember how thrilled I was. I think I just wanted the diagnostic team to know that Jonah wasn't disengaged from the world, completely isolated behind an impenetrable wall. I kept thinking of Helen Keller before Annie Sullivan taught her language. That one sign gave me so much hope. I wanted the team to know, as I knew, that not only did Jonah want some of the same things as typical children did, but he was able to ask for them. Not that his sign staved off the expected autism diagnosis, because that's exactly what he got—not even the trendy PDD/NOS (pervasive developmental disorder/not otherwise specified) diagnosis, otherwise known as "autism lite," that was becoming popular with doctors who either felt their young patients didn't meet all the criteria of autism or who, in many cases, were just trying to cushion the blow for devastated parents.

One big difference between this trip to Mount Sinai and our drive to CHOP so long ago is that Jonah isn't with us. It would be nearly impossible for us to keep him confined in an office for any length of time, so this exploratory meeting with Dr. Kellner is just for Andy and me—which lends the ride a bizarrely festive air. A night away from the kids is pretty rare for us, and I'm particularly relishing the possibility of eight uninterrupted hours of sleep. Not only does Jonah routinely get up at four or five in the morning—after which he sometimes goes back to sleep, but more often is up for the day—but the twins, at three-and-a-half, are not past their own occasional midnight visits. Gretchen especially is prone to nightmares. Last week she came crying into our room sometime around two thirty, and when I pressed her to tell me about her bad dream, she sobbed, "I dreamed I gave Aaron candy and I told him not to eat it, but he ate it anyway!"

We're staying at the apartment Andy shared with a co-worker for the better part of the past year, during which he commuted back and forth to New York. He hasn't used it much since his company opened a new office five minutes from our home in Pennsylvania, but the lovely pied à terre only contributes to the holiday mood. Andy needs to go into the office tomorrow before our eleven o'clock appointment, but I'm looking forward to a morning of sleeping in, then a stroll to Starbucks, where I intend to drink myself dizzy on their darkest roast while finally making a dent in the pile of ECT papers—some from Dr. Wachtel, others I've found myself online—I've only managed to skim through since our conversation two-and-a-half weeks ago.

Until the phone rings at six thirty, thwarting at least the first part of my plan. It's Keri, calling to ask me about Jonah's new iTouch, which we had to replace because Jonah dropped the first one in the toilet—accidentally, we presume, but we may be giving him too much credit. Did I load Jonah's videos before I left? I thought I had, I tell her, but she says that when Jonah tries to play one, no titles are listed. I realize immediately that, in my haste to leave for New York, I must have unplugged the iTouch from the computer before it was done downloading all Jonah's movies and music.

"Just plug the Touch into my—" I start, then realize my laptop is ten feet away from me, not back on my desk at home. "Oh, no."

This is why it's hard for us to be away. Because when something goes wrong, it has the potential to explode into catastrophe: *What will Jonah do without his iTouch?* That little video player has proven to be a real lifesaver—it's gotten us through interminable traffic jams, long lines at Costco, and the daily forty minute rides to and from school, which used to be so distressing to Jonah he would pound on the windows, hit the aide, and kick the seats enough to earn us a repair bill from the transport company—but on the flip side, he's definitely grown dependent on it. Will he throw a tantrum? Will he go after Keri when she tells him she can't fix it? How will he get through the ride to school? I feel absolutely terrible to have put Keri in this position—how could I not have double-checked? Keri tells me not to worry about it—she'll figure something out.

I hang up but am unable to go back to sleep. After lying in bed for a few minutes, I give up and take a shower. The shower in that apartment is the hottest, hardest shower I've ever been in, and I stand under it for half an hour—my cell phone perched on the edge of the sink in case there are any other problems at home. But it doesn't ring, and when I call Keri back after I'm dressed she tells me that she managed to find a Sesame Street video on iTunes that Jonah seemed to find acceptable. "Everything's fine," she says. "Good luck with your meeting."

I spend the rest of the morning as I had originally planned, holed up in Starbucks reading ECT studies before meeting Andy for the cab ride uptown. I've come across Dr. Kellner's name many times in my research—he's a major figure in the field and has authored over a hundred fifty articles, examining everything from electrode placement to societal perceptions of ECT to cognitive effects. He was also inducted—involuntarily, of course—into the anti-ECT organization ect.org's "Hall of Shame" for his efforts. Given how he has loomed larger than life in my imagination, I have to hide my surprise when the man himself steps out of his office to shake our hands: somehow, I expected him to be . . . larger. Slight, with a grizzled beard, there's something almost Ben Kingsley-like about both his features and his quiet gravitas. I trust him immediately.

Dr. Kellner invites us to sit down and starts asking us about Jonah's history in his soft, even voice. My eyes drift to the certificates and diplomas hanging on the walls. Jonah, I muse, couldn't be further removed from Dr. Kellner's typical patients—he's a geriatric psychiatrist, as are many doctors who perform ECT. This makes sense, given the demographics: studies have found that more than 50 percent of ECT patients are over sixty. The elderly suffer from depression—the most common diagnosis for which ECT is prescribed—at a much higher rate than their younger cohorts. They also present a greater suicide risk, making a fast-acting agent like ECT preferable to antidepressants, which can take several weeks to work, if they work at all, and are often poorly tolerated by this population anyway.[1]

Dr. Kellner's specialty may make him seem a poor match for Jonah, but we aren't the first family to turn to him for assistance. Those other children, just like Jonah, were referred by colleagues who believed ECT was indicated but couldn't offer it themselves due to restrictions imposed by their states or hospitals. Despite the fact that Philadelphia, where we live, is home to many of the nation's top hospitals, several of which offer ECT through their psychiatric departments, Dr. Wachtel couldn't think of one local doctor who would agree to provide ECT to a patient as young as Jonah.

"Have you thought about whether we should do the ECT on an inpatient or outpatient basis?" Dr. Kellner asks. We had discussed this briefly on the phone: although patients are often admitted for the initial course of ECT, Dr. Kellner had told me it would be easier to get Jonah accepted as a patient if we could do it on an outpatient basis—the pediatric unit at Mount Sinai just isn't equipped, as the NBU is, to handle kids with extreme behaviors.

"We can do outpatient," I say, even though it means we'll have to get Jonah to New York by seven a.m. three times a week for approximately three weeks. The hedge fund Andy works for is headquartered in Manhattan; he says he will trade out of that office those days, so I won't have to make the drive—which can take five hours or more, roundtrip—by myself. The good news is that Dr. Kellner has a colleague at a psychiatric facility twenty minutes away from us, whom he suspects could be persuaded to perform maintenance ECT on Jonah if the acute course is successful.

It's a relief to hear we won't have to commute to Mount Sinai forever, but still surprising that there's only one practice in the fifth largest city in the country that *might* treat my son. Maybe I shouldn't be so surprised: as controversial as ECT is, it's even more controversial when used on children, and more controversial still when used on children with intellectual disabilities. After all, such patients are the most vulnerable, the most in need of protection. But they are also often the ones most in need of help. Kitty Dukakis describes in the book *Shock: The Healing Power of Electroconvulsive Therapy* that thanks to her first sessions of ECT her chronic depression finally lifted, allowing her to "eat out at a restaurant that night. . . . After the second one I went to the hairdresser, then a dinner party." I don't mean to belittle anyone's suffering—believe me, I know the social, intellectual and emotional impairments endemic to mental illness can be profoundly debilitating. But for children with aggressive, self-injurious, and catatonic symptoms, the stakes are exponentially higher. The parents I spoke to as Andy and I considered ECT for Jonah firmly believe their kids (some of whose stories are included here) would be blind, institutionalized, or dead without it.

Five states—California, Colorado, Louisiana, Tennessee, and Texas—prohibit the use of ECT on children under any circumstances, although my research found no evidence that ECT is harmful to developing brains. Minors represent only a tiny fraction of the millions of people who have been treated with ECT since it was first introduced in 1938—one 1987 paper estimated that 500 to 3,500 of the 100,000 Americans who receive ECT each year are between the ages of eleven and twenty.[2] Another offered the much higher estimate of one percent of all ECT patients worldwide, hypothesizing that the greater popularity of ECT in developing countries, such as India, may account for the difference.[3]

Despite its infrequent use in juveniles, doctors have been examining the safety and efficacy of ECT in treating serious mental illness in this population for almost sixty years. The largest and one of the oldest reports of ECT in children is the infamous 1947 study at Bellevue Hospital. Dr. Lauretta Bender administered ECT six times a week to ninety-eight kids who all had been diagnosed with acute schizophrenia, the youngest only four and none older than eleven. Anti-ECT activists have a field day with this study, as you might imagine. They point out that few of these young patients would meet today's criteria for childhood schizophrenia, which is true: a follow-up study in 1954 that included thirty-two of the patients previously treated at Bellevue found that most of the children actually suffered from behavior disorders or psychopathic personalities. And these kids had nothing positive to say about their experience with ECT: one nine-year-old boy tried to hang himself because he was afraid of additional treatments, and another boy, Ted Chabasinski, has spent his adult life lobbying for the abolition of ECT. None of this is particularly astonishing, given that the children in Bender's study were given unmodified ECT—the general anesthesia, oxygenation, and muscle relaxants used today didn't catch on until the mid-1950s. Of course, this would be a terrifying experience for young kids; as Chabasinski remembers, "They would stick a rag in my mouth so I wouldn't bite through my tongue and it took three attendants to hold me down."[4] But it's also not hard to understand why Bender was so interested in how her young patients would respond to ECT—in 1947, there were few options available for mentally ill patients of any age. Those who didn't respond to psychotherapy—and there were many—often faced a lifetime of institutionalization. Before the FDA approved Thorazine in 1954, launching an avalanche of new psychotropic medications, psychiatrists used ECT much more indiscriminately than they do today because it was the only treatment that ever worked.[5]

Despite its limitations, there are still important takeaways from the Bender study. Most significant is Bender's findings on cognitive impairment following ECT. From the very beginning, doctors have been concerned about the effect of ECT on young brains. Bender was careful to administer a battery of tests to her patients before and after their treatments. She reported, "The psychological tests are further characterized by lack of any evidence for a lasting effect on the intellectual functioning and development of the child as a result of the electric shock, although five children showed some interference in function immediately after treatment."[6] Even the critical follow-up study out of Rockland State Hospital confirmed that "follow-up psychometric testing disclosed no significant deviations from the preshock levels of intellectual functioning."[7]

This same pattern, cognitive impairments directly following ECT that resolved to pre-ECT levels of performance or better, was also reported in two 1947 articles by different research teams.[8] More than fifty years later, two French studies compared adolescents who had received ECT with peers with the same diagnoses who had been treated instead with psychotropic medication. One study tested ten subjects an average of three and a half years after treatment; the other followed up eleven patients a little over five years later.[9] Both groups were indistinguishable from controls in their cognitive scores, social functioning, and academic achievement. In 2000, doctors at the University of Michigan tested sixteen teenagers with mood disorders before, immediately after, and eight months following their acute courses of ECT; although their patients did score lower on tests of attention and concentration conducted one week post-ECT, the researchers found that "eight months following ECT treatment, subjects did not differ significantly from baseline levels."[10] Most recently, a Japanese study of ECT on young adults with schizophrenia also found no difference on cognitive tests given pre- and post-treatment.[11]

So Andy and I aren't afraid that ECT will have any permanent effects on Jonah's uncanny, innate reading ability, or on the math skills he's managed to acquire despite spending half his school days in time-out. The cognitive function most at risk, ECT experts agree, is memory.

"Jonah probably won't remember much from the three-month period surrounding the acute course of ECT," Dr. Kellner warns us. I nod: we already know. This position—that ECT causes only mild and restricted memory loss, if any—is shared by the great majority of practitioners, as well as the most prominent figures who have spoken publicly about their positive experiences with ECT. These include Kitty Dukakis, psychotherapist and author Martha Manning, and Dr. Sherwin B. Nuland, who credits ECT with saving him from the lobotomy that his doctors had determined was the only recourse left to break the incapacitating depression with which he was hospitalized in his early forties. Far from suffering any cognitive impairments, Dr. Nuland was able to resume his surgical practice and went on to write nine books, including the National Book Award-winning *How We Die*.

But this position is by no means unanimous. There are many "survivors" who maintain they lost several years of their lives to ECT. And in 2005, former patient Peggy Salters was awarded over $600,000 after suing her psychiatrist for referring her for ECT based on her claim that it had wiped out over thirty years' worth of memories, including those of her husband, who had since died, and the births of her three children.

But memory loss is tough to evaluate. Anecdotal accounts flourish in support groups and on the Internet, but as Dr. Max Fink argues in a paper published in the journal *Psychosomatics*, other factors are often at play. Brutal media depictions of ECT, passionate claims by "survivors," and even the consent forms patients are required to sign prior to ECT all make it easy to attribute gaps in memory to ECT, even though age, mental illness itself, anesthesia, and the natural lapses in memory everyone experiences are all potential culprits.[12] An additional complicating factor is that most patients with mental illness have been prescribed many different drugs over the course of their illnesses that can also wreak havoc with memory. Benzodiazepines (i.e., Valium), for example, don't erase memories of the past so much as they may prevent current experiences from being encoded into long-term memory—a phenomenon known as anterograde amnesia.

Still, anti-ECT activists lit up the web in 2007 when psychologist Dr. Harold Sackeim published a study that, according to Linda Andre, one of the most vocal "survivors" writing on ect.org, conceded for the first time that "ECT routinely causes permanent memory loss and deficits in cognitive abilities." But this statement simply isn't true, not in its depiction of the psychiatric profession's approach to ECT in general or of this study's findings in particular. First of all, doctors have long acknowledged that patients often experience short-term amnesia following ECT. In its 1985 Consensus Statement on Electroconvulsive Therapy, twenty-two years before Dr. Sackeim's study, the National Institutes of Health—while endorsing the use of ECT to treat certain severe mental illnesses, including depression and bipolar disorder—stated in no uncertain terms, "Deficits in memory function, which have been demonstrated objectively and repeatedly, persist after the termination of a normal course of ECT."[13]

So Dr. Sackeim's report of memory loss was hardly news. Furthermore, it's not even clear how much amnesia his subjects really experienced. What he found was that, six months after ECT, patients scored worse than controls on the AMI-SF, a test of autobiographical memory. But these results are difficult to interpret. First of all, this test was designed by Dr. Sackeim's own group and has never been independently validated—a fact which, interestingly, has caused zealots on both sides of the ECT debate to reject it. Even assuming the test measures what it claims to measure, the bulk of the questions concern recent events: each subject is asked to recall details of her last vacation, doctor visit, and birthday, among other things. It's very likely that the subjects in the ECT group were being asked to remember at least some events well within the period of amnesia that, as Dr. Kellner warned us about, generally clouds the months surrounding the acute course of ECT. Second, and more importantly, it's impossible to determine from the article exactly how much memory loss the ECT group actually suffered. Dr. Sackeim wrote that, at the six-month follow-up, "The average decrement in AMI-SF scores in patients treated with BL ECT was . . . 2.8 times the amount of forgetting seen in the healthy comparison groups."[14] But what does this mean? How many more of the thirty questions on the test did they miss? I asked Dr. Sackeim to provide this additional information, but he declined to share his data. It certainly seems unlikely the control group would forget many of the details they had been asked to provide only six months before, which means the difference in the groups could amount to little more than one or two questions.

But there's no doubt that the scarier part of Andre's claim is her pronouncement that the subjects in Dr. Sackeim's study—and by extrapolation, ECT patients in general—suffered "deficits in cognitive abilities." I have no idea how Andre arrived at this interpretation, since Dr. Sackeim is clear that he found quite the opposite. Although his patients did perform worse on some tests immediately following ECT, which is typical, Dr. Sackeim clearly wrote, "most cognitive parameters were substantially improved at six-month follow-up relative to pre-ECT baseline, presumably because of the negative impact of the depressed state on baseline performance." Those parameters included measures of attention, learning ability, and global cognitive status—which, in other words, were all *higher* post-ECT compared to initial scores.

Furthermore, Dr. Sackeim did convincingly show that techno-logical developments designed to reduce the negative cognitive side effects of ECT have done exactly that. Originally, ECT was per-formed with the type of current that comes out of a wall socket, called a sine wave. Although clinicians began to turn to an alterna-tive waveform known as "brief pulse" as early as the mid-twentieth century (with current research focusing on an even lighter variant, "ultra brief-pulse"), a small minority of hospitals still uses sine waves today. Dr. Sackeim and his colleagues compared test scores of patients from different hospitals and confirmed that those who received sine wave stimulation exhibited "more severe short-term memory deficits" as well as impairments in psychomotor response speed, which is probably why the American Psychiatric Association declared in 2001 that "the continued use of sine wave stimulation in ECT is not justified."[15]

I don't mean to suggest that everyone who blames ECT for signifi-cant amnesia is faking it, because that's not what I believe. I read with great sympathy Jonathan Cott's meditation *On the Sea of Memory: A Journey from Forgetting to Remembering* in which he describes the dev-astating loss of fifteen years of memories following the ECT he was given in 1998 to treat his debilitating depression and suicidal idea-tion. But I do agree with neurobiologist James L. McGaugh, whom Cott quotes in his own book: "That would be unusual for ECT to have such an effect." Although I'm sure knowing he is part of a very small minority doesn't make Cott feel any better, the fact remains that because no medical procedure is completely free of side effects, patients must always consider the risks before choosing a course of treatment. Chemotherapy, radiation, anti-epileptic medication, and cardiac surgery, like ECT, can also have cognitive side effects; a 2001 study in *The New England Journal of Medicine* found that more than 40 percent of patients who underwent bypass surgery showed cogni-tive deficits of 20 percent or more five years later.[16] Yet no activists lobby Congress to ban these treatments; no bloggers compare the doctors who perform them to Nazis; no concerned citizens suggest that patients suffering from cancer or angina not undergo these life-saving therapies.

Our hopes for ECT are no less profound than those other patients invest in bypass surgery or cancer treatment. When I ask Dr. Kellner how much of an improvement we can expect to see in Jonah following ECT, he asks me about the best Jonah has ever behaved. I immediately think back to one of our last visits to Kennedy Krieger when Andy and I took Jonah to a supermarket along with one of his behavioral therapists. Jonah's obsession with food triggers a significant percentage of his outbursts, so we were asking a lot from him: to help us buy everything on our shopping list—which consisted entirely of the chips, candy, and other edibles the therapists on the NBU used as reinforcers with their patients—without getting one treat for himself. I wouldn't even expect this from my other children, whom I usually reward with at least a small snack for accompanying me on my most tedious errands and who have far fewer problems with frustration and impulse control than Jonah. It wasn't as if he didn't want anything, because he asked constantly: "Blue juice?" (Gatorade); "White chips?" (salt and vinegar potato chips); "Jellybeans, Skittles, Mike & Ikes, fruit snacks, marshmallows?" But we told him no, we re-directed him back to the list, and he was fine. No tantrums, no grabbing, no dashing across the store at full speed to stick his finger in a sheet cake (which has happened more than once). His medication was perfectly calibrated, so instead of presenting as a simmering cauldron of agitation threatening to boil over at any moment, as I often see him, Jonah radiated a real sense of peace.

When I tell Dr. Kellner this story, he says that degree of mood stability is exactly what he would expect from ECT. And this will save Jonah's life—at least, his quality of life. He will still be autistic, of course—ECT won't help the social and linguistic impairments typical of spectrum disorders. I know Jonah won't start chatting about his days or asking for play dates like my other kids. But Dr. Wachtel has always believed Jonah's aggressive and self-injurious behaviors were primarily functions of his bipolar disorder, and mood disorders like bipolar and depression respond very well to ECT. If Jonah can be trusted not to hit I'll be able to take him anywhere by myself. He'll be able to continue to do the things he loves to do: eat at Burger King, peruse the video selection at Best Buy, go to the beach, stroll the boardwalk in Atlantic City—things that right now he can only do with Andy, who can still manage Jonah's most explosive outbursts, but soon may not be able to do at all.

So for us, as for all patients considering ECT, it comes down to a cost-benefit analysis. No doubt, Jonah will experience some memory loss—in all likelihood, just the brief period Dr. Kellner described. Possibly, it could be more. But honestly, Jonah doesn't have much to remember. His behaviors have so restricted his activities that he's never done Little League or acted in a play. His last vacation, aside from our regular trips to our house in Atlantic City, was almost five years ago because I've been too scared to take him on a plane. The place that he most asks to go back to, hilariously enough, is the NBU. Even though he was on a locked ward, even though the food was terrible, the patients were loud, and he had to share a room with three or sometimes four other boys, he still misses the great therapists and aides who really loved him—so much so that, a year later, I'm still getting emails from them asking how he's doing. The fact is, ECT is the best chance Jonah has to celebrate the kind of milestones people remember most: a bar mitzvah, a graduation, a first job. For us, given the alternatives—or rather, the lack thereof—the choice is obvious.

But making the choice isn't enough. New York State requires the approval of two independent psychiatrists before ECT is permitted; Dr. Kellner tells us he will have to convene a meeting of the ethics committee. And it so happens that the committee has just accepted another of Dr. Wachtel's referrals, a patient who was admitted to Mount Sinai last week. The easy approval is a good sign, but Dr. Kellner can't bring another patient before the committee so soon. We will have to wait and see how this other patient responds. Compounding the delay is the impending Christmas holiday, but Dr. Kellner expresses his hope as we leave that Jonah will able to start ECT as early as January.

CHAPTER 2

Matthew

Stepping into Tom and Cheryl's minivan was déjà vu for me: *Sesame Street* music on the CD player, the Kennedy Krieger Institute looming behind us, and a pale, dark-haired boy under a blanket in the back seat, snuggled next to his mother. It could have been me and Jonah during one of our many visits to Baltimore over the course of his ten-month hospitalization. But this time it was another boy I had come to visit: Tom and Cheryl's thirteen-year-old son, Matthew, who was admitted to KKI's Neurobehavioral Unit (NBU) in March 2009, like Jonah, for uncontrollable aggressive and self-injurious behaviors (SIBs).

We were well on our way to McDonald's—also a favorite of Jonah's—before Matthew emerged from his blanket to check me out. Diagnosed with autism and mental retardation, Matthew is non-verbal. Instead of greeting me vocally, he smiled, and that's when I noticed his eyes, which weren't like Jonah's at all. Not only are Matthew's eyes a striking grey-green color, but there was something subtly asymmetrical about his gaze that took me a moment to pinpoint: Matthew's right pupil was much more dilated than his left. This, I learned, was because the lens in his right eye had been removed during surgery ten months ago. Matthew's SIB was so bad that he had detached his own retinas.

Tom and Cheryl weren't even sure when the injury occurred, but it was diagnosed during routine tests KKI performs on all new patients who bang or hit themselves on the head. Matthew, who, at the time of his admission, hit himself in the face an average of two hundred times *every hour*, clearly met those criteria. Ophthalmologists estimated the retinas had been detached for at least three, and possibly five, months. Tom and Cheryl were shocked; because Matthew

---

All names have been changed to protect privacy.

doesn't speak, he couldn't even tell them how badly his vision had deteriorated. Surgery was required immediately.

Tom and Cheryl's planned four-day trip to Baltimore to help Matthew settle in at KKI stretched to forty days. Although the surgery went well, Matthew detached his right retina a second time within a week. His doctors agreed to a second surgery, but warned that Matthew would blind himself unless his SIB could be stopped—something eight previous hospitalizations and a year in a residential treatment facility had failed to do. It was at this point that Dr. Wachtel, Matthew's new psychiatrist at KKI, suggested he might be a good candidate for ECT.

Tom and Cheryl aren't the kind of parents who blindly follow their doctors. They have been integrally involved in Matthew's treatment since he was diagnosed at twenty-one months. Tom even stepped down from his managerial position with an insurance company to take a more supportive role, one that would allow him to work fewer and more flexible hours, so he could focus on Matthew's care. Tom and Cheryl designed spreadsheets charting every medication Matthew has ever taken, the dosages prescribed, and their effects—or, in many cases, the lack thereof—and have chronicled every specialist their son has seen, every diagnostic test, every hospitalization. While Matthew was still living at home, Tom and Cheryl were in constant contact with the school district, as well as the agencies that provided their home aides. When they found a residential treatment program they thought might help their son, they fought to create a new state funding program to support children as young as Matthew (then eight) in residential placements if their conditions warranted it. Six months later, when they decided it wasn't helping, they marshaled all the state and local agencies required to bring him home.

So, when Dr. Wachtel and Matthew's NBU team recommended ECT, Tom and Cheryl didn't agree immediately. They ordered a book on ECT to be delivered overnight to their hotel and spent the weekend reading it, along with any articles they could find on the Internet. They spoke personally with the doctor who would be performing the ECT. Only when they felt sufficiently educated did Cheryl give their answer: "How soon can we start?"

"It was a no-brainer," Cheryl said, as we waited in a booth at

McDonald's for Tom to navigate the overloaded tray to our table—including two fish sandwiches for Matthew, who was understandably compensating for a week's worth of tasteless hospital fare. With Matthew's eyesight on the line and his poor track record with psychotropics, Tom and Cheryl didn't want to waste time with another medication. Since the age of three Matthew had been prescribed thirty-eight different medications that spanned the entire pharmacological spectrum: antipsychotics, antidepressants, anticonvulsants, antihypertensives, mood stabilizers, and stimulants. Each seemed to have more bizarre side effects than the last. One gave Matthew painful erections that lasted an hour or more. Another made it nearly impossible for him to swallow; he lost more than fifteen pounds in a matter of weeks. "My sister brought over a dozen donuts, Matthew's favorite," Cheryl remembered. "He chewed up the entire box while leaning over a trash can, spitting out every bite."

Alternative remedies touted by some members of the autism community had been similarly unsuccessful. Tom and Cheryl put Matthew on a gluten- and casein-free diet, infused him with Secretin, and dosed him with probiotics, vitamins, fish oil, and flaxseed oil—none of which helped at all. Even if the safety and efficacy of ECT hadn't been established to their satisfaction by more than half a century of scientific studies, the simple truth remained, as Tom said, "There was nothing else to try."

Matthew was given ECT three times before his second surgery, but his ophthalmologists didn't dare wait any longer to reattach the right retina. This time, the surgical team wasn't taking any chances: they put Matthew in a medically-induced coma for seven days to give his eye a better opportunity to heal. Tom and Cheryl stayed with him throughout, trying to comfort him any way they could as the extended anesthesia took its toll. Matthew suffered a collapsed lung, pneumonia, persistent diarrhea, and chafing on his face from the foam supports that stabilized him in the prone position in which he spent twenty hours out of every day. Hanging over them was the fear that this would happen again as soon as Matthew regained consciousness. He was scheduled to resume his ECT as soon as he was discharged from the ICU, but how long would the treatments take to work? What if they didn't work?

When Matthew returned to the NBU, he was fitted with a helmet as well as arm restraints to keep him from bending his elbows. Every waking moment there were four aides assigned to make sure that he never ever hit himself in the face. Tom and Cheryl, who still couldn't bring themselves to leave Baltimore and return to their home almost four hundred miles away, couldn't even get close to their son, he was so tightly guarded. Matthew received ECT three times a week, and after each session, his parents examined him closely, trying to determine if his behavior was any better. The restraints, the staffing, these weren't long-term solutions. ECT had to work. The alternative—a life of institutionalization, blindness, stuporous sedation—was too grim to consider. Which meant, naturally, that they dwelled on it constantly.

————

One drawback about life on the NBU is that the kids don't get outside much. Even though it was a frigid twenty-five degrees, Tom and Cheryl wanted Matthew to get some fresh air. They bundled him up and we drove to a beautiful playground, completely deserted under the January sunshine. Tom and Matthew climbed for a few minutes, then we fed a flock of well-mannered geese who were thrilled to see us and our leftover French fries. It wasn't long before the cold drove us back to the car. We decided to go to the Whitemarsh Mall, where Tom and Matthew rode the same carousel Andy and I had ridden with our kids on many of our weekly trips to Baltimore (there's only so many times you can visit the Inner Harbor). Cheryl and I waved as they went past.

"We could never do this before ECT," Cheryl said, with an expansive wave that included the carousel, the mall, McDonald's. "There would be pickles on the ceiling." She glanced around. "Matthew would rip that sign off the wall. We couldn't take him anywhere. He would just flip out, all the time." It was hard for me to imagine, even though I knew better than most what those rages looked like. Matthew hung on his mother's arm while we strolled the mall, taking a few extra turns on the escalator, just for fun. Not once during the entire afternoon did he hit himself or anyone else. He just seemed happy to be spending time with his parents.

Tom and Cheryl abandoned many dreams along the journey that has been their life together. Both from large families, Tom initially told Cheryl he wanted "eleven children—an entire football team."

But after ten years of trying, including two on Clomid, they only had one. Neither Matthew's autism nor Cheryl's difficult pregnancy—suffering from hyper-emesis, she lost thirty-five pounds over the course of the pregnancy—discouraged them from attempting to give Matthew a sibling. It wasn't until Cheryl had a miscarriage after her fourth IVF attempt that she and Tom decided to focus all their attention on Matthew.

As the scope of Matthew's impairment became evident, Tom and Cheryl tried to keep their expectations low. Determined to be realistic, they didn't want to be the kind of parents who stubbornly cling to goals their children would never meet. There was one dream they wouldn't relinquish, however: they wanted their son to be happy. But happy hardly described Matthew's life in the years prior to his admission to KKI.

"Since he was five, I think Matthew's been in the hospital more than he's been home," Cheryl told me over chai lattés we picked up at Starbucks after taking Matthew back to KKI (patients aren't allowed to be off the unit for more than four hours at a time). Not that any of Matthew's eight hospitalizations helped much. Although improved at discharge, shortly after returning home, Matthew's behavior inevitably deteriorated once again. He was prone to frequent bouts of unprovoked aggression, including biting, kicking, hitting, pinching, hair-pulling, and spitting. There were times when Cheryl was alone with Matthew that she had to lock herself in the bathroom while he pounded on the door, trying to attack her. And his retinal re-attachment wasn't the first operation necessitated by his severe SIB: Matthew also needed surgery to repair a bite to his hand and another to treat hematomas on both ears. Too unmanageable to take out in the community—Tom and Cheryl's last car had big bites in the upholstery and dents in the rear panels from one disastrous outing—Matthew only left the house to go to school. Sometimes, he didn't even make it that far. Tom and Cheryl had to home-school Matthew for periods when even his specialized autistic support program couldn't handle him.

Still, Tom and Cheryl never gave up their dream of happiness for their son. When his world shrank to the confines of their home they did whatever they could to bring Matthew's favorite activities to him. Maybe they could no longer take him sailing or skating, but since Matthew loves swimming, his parents bought an above-ground pool—and installed a six-foot high stockade fence around the perimeter of their yard so Matthew wouldn't bolt into the street while he was outside enjoying it. He loves camping, so Tom set up their tent and lit campfires in their backyard. "We would hear Matthew at eleven o'clock at night, grabbing the hot dogs from the refrigerator and my guitar from the basement, because he wanted another campfire," Tom said.

But as Matthew entered adolescence, he became so persistently agitated that not even his pool or campfires made him happy. His behavior kept worsening, while the time home between admissions kept shrinking. Matthew's last hospitalization before KKI came only ten days after his discharge from the same facility. Tom and Cheryl were called by Matthew's teacher to come to school immediately; an ambulance was on its way for Matthew, who was so out-of-control it required six adults to restrain him. Although doctors hadn't come up with any new ideas since the previous week when they had sent Matthew home, they agreed to keep him until a bed opened up at KKI. It took seven long months, during which the hospitals were in constant contact, for Matthew to be transferred.

————

Fortunately, Tom and Cheryl didn't have to wait long to see an effect from ECT. Three weeks after his second retinal reattachment, the ophthalmologist observed that Matthew seemed much calmer. He had been able to lie down for a check of his intraocular pressure that involved placing an instrument directly on his eyeball, a procedure that had previously required restraints.

Over the next five months, Matthew's ECT schedule was thinned, from three times a week, to twice, to weekly, then to biweekly treatments. In February 2010, ten months after his first ECT and almost two months after I had met him in Baltimore, Matthew was discharged from KKI. His rate of aggression had dropped 77 percent; his SIB was reduced by 98 percent. His behavior wasn't perfect—he still had trouble hearing "no" or "wait"—but his tantrums were both less frequent and less intense, and his team at KKI had designed a behavior plan to address these lingering issues.

Tom and Cheryl saw no evidence of side effects from the fifty-six ECT treatments Matthew received while at KKI. Although some critics claim that ECT leaves patients apathetic and little more than emotionless zombies, Tom and Cheryl reported the opposite was true: Matthew was more engaged since he started ECT, his receptive language seemed to have improved, and he followed directions better. "Last week, Matthew finished his dinner and signed 'done' without any prompting for the very first time," Tom told me, the day I visited them in Baltimore. "Usually, we have to ask over and over, 'Are you done?' and if he doesn't push his food away, we assume he's not done. Seeing him sign on his own like that, I almost cried."

The biggest concern, when a child is discharged from KKI, is maintaining the gains made while there. When Jonah came home, the insurance company that picked up the bill for his hospitalization on behalf of the State of Pennsylvania hired a renowned psychologist and author of eight books on behavioral intervention to assist in his transition. The psychologist told me that patients often relapse to some degree after leaving the highly controlled environment of the NBU—which did in fact happen to Jonah. But three years after Matthew's discharge, he was still stable, still living at home—his longest stretch without a hospitalization since he was five years old. He recently moved from a very small private school for autistic children to an autism support program in the public high school, where Tom felt he enjoyed interacting with other students. There, in addition to the typical Applied Behavior Analysis (ABA) drills ubiquitous in autism classrooms, Matthew had the opportunity to take wood shop and volunteer at a food bank where he packed boxes. A more important development Tom shared with me early in 2013 was that Matthew's team was teaching him to communicate with an iPad. "Right now, it's still very basic; he's just requesting things that he wants, like his favorite snacks, or a drink, or the bathroom," Tom said. "When Matthew wants something, he taps the picture and the iPad also speaks for him." Before ECT, he would have thrown the device across the room. Now, Matthew will finally have a voice.

Outside of school, Tom explained, "Things are pretty routine for us now"—an unremarkable statement that, given the family's history, was profoundly remarkable. Matthew likes to hike, do puzzles, and listen to his father play the guitar. "When I play, he goes around and shuts all the lights off," Tom said. "He likes it completely dark. And he will come and lie beside me and listen sometimes for an hour. Matthew is always on the move, so this is unique." Tom wrote several songs for Matthew, including one about his son's absolute favorite activity. "It's called 'I Just Want to Go for a Ride.' It's basically about Matthew not caring about anything except going for a ride. It's a fast tune," he explained. Their seven-month-old car, he added, already had almost 10,000 miles on it—and not one bite mark.

Although Matthew was discharged from KKI on a biweekly maintenance schedule, his parents and his doctors discovered that his stability was maximized with weekly ECT. As of February 2013, he has had 238 treatments—which he doesn't seem to find aversive. When they arrive at the hospital, Matthew jumps up on the gurney and pulls down the nitrous oxide mask, anticipating every step of the process. Cheryl thinks that, somehow, he understands that ECT makes him feel better.

It certainly helped get through puberty, which as I mentioned earlier is typically a very difficult time for autistic boys, during which aggressive and self-injurious behaviors can be greatly exacerbated. Matthew was the only other boy I knew—besides Jonah—who began ECT before puberty, so I was greatly interested to discover whether its stabilizing effects had prevented the behavioral deterioration often precipitated by the hormonal frenzy experienced by all adolescents.

"We did have to teach Matthew that some things are only OK to do in the privacy of your own room," Cheryl explained to me tactfully when I saw her at a meeting at KKI. "Sometimes he just bolts off the school bus, drops his backpack by the front door, and runs up to his room and slams the door." I laughed, relieved that the worst part of Matthew's puberty was his intense interest in masturbation—an obsession, I was reasonably certain, shared by most neurotypical teenage boys.

For Tom, his son's experience with ECT has been nothing short of life changing. "All the typical dreams went out the window the day Matthew was diagnosed," he said. But recently, he's begun imagining a future for Matthew that involves friends, independence, maybe a job. He and Cheryl have even considered buying the house next door and turning it into a group home where Matthew and a few developmentally delayed peers could live with the appropriate support—although they debate whether Cheryl could resist constantly checking on the young men if they were so close. "A few of those dreams," Tom admitted, "a few are coming back now."

CHAPTER 3

Jonah,
January-March 2010
THE EFFICACY STUDIES

JANUARY THROUGH MID-FEBRUARY 2010

We wait.

We wait through the long Christmas break, with no school and no aides. Andy had intended to take this week off, but his fund is busier than anticipated and he can only get away for a few half-days. I know all the museums and indoor play spaces will be packed because of the holiday, and we can't even go to the zoo—our favorite winter destination since it's so empty this time of year—because it's bitterly cold. In the end, we spend a lot of time at home.

It makes me feel petty when I long to be able to take my family on vacation. It seems like such a superficial thing to waste my energy thinking about when I should be focused on executing Jonah's behavior plan as well as humanly possible, while spending enough time with my other four kids so they don't decide they love the nannies more than me: I fail at both routinely. And self-pity is such an ugly emotion. I try to ease my guilt by assuring myself that this kind of escapism is perfectly normal, that there's nothing wrong with dreaming about a few days in the sun when it's twenty degrees outside. I know that what I really crave isn't the sun so much as it is the ease with which my friends and their families can hop on a plane and go . . . anywhere.

I'm sure I sound about as sympathetic as Leona Helmsley, whining that I can't go on vacation while most of the world struggles just to get by. But in truth, not a day passes that I'm not profoundly grateful for our financial security. Keri and I grew up with very little; our parents divorced when I was seven, and because my father was sick the rest of his life, my mother supported us on her secretary's salary. Until I was thirteen, we lived in a dim basement apartment so persis-

31

tently infested with bugs that it took years for me to lose the reflex I had developed of automatically pausing a few seconds after opening a drawer to let the roaches scurry out of the light. I feel very lucky to be able to give my own kids so many things I didn't have. But even more than that, I feel very lucky to be able to provide Jonah with everything he needs. I'm sure there are problems in the world that can't be solved by throwing a lot of money at them, but caring for a child with a developmental disability isn't one of them. I'm constantly thankful we can afford aides, private camps, alternative therapies, specialists, prescriptions, and educational materials. Once when Jonah was much younger Andy made a comment I never forgot, mainly because I never considered him to be particularly spiritual: "If God looks over the world, searching for the right homes for kids with special needs, we were a good choice." And he didn't mean because we're especially selfless or patient—because I assure you, we're not.

Besides, it isn't at all a fancy resort that I long for. Even the tropical climate is entirely optional. What would be really nice, the only vacation that would really make a difference for me, would be one from this constant vigilance, the need to always be watching Jonah's ever-vacillating moods, anticipating what might provoke an outburst (which could be anything, or nothing), and planning ahead how to contain it safely. The need for a vacation from that ever-present hitch at the back of my throat that is sometimes very hard to distinguish from resentment. Which, naturally, brings the guilt crashing back down, starting the cycle all over again.

Periodically, I email Dr. Kellner. I don't want to nag, but I really want to know—especially as the January days tick by—what the heck is taking so long? That's not what I write in my emails, of course. I write, "I was wondering if you had any updates." I write, "Just checking in." I write, "Thank you so much for all your help." And Dr. Kellner writes back that his current patient is improving, but slowly. He writes, "I can assure you that not a day goes by when [Jonah] is not on my mind (several times)."

There's nothing more frustrating than knowing there's something out there that doctors you trust believe will likely ease your child's suffering and not being able to try it NOW: not because it's too expensive, or too far away, but because of politics. I understand that Dr. Kellner must be sensitive to the political climate at Mount Sinai or we run the risk of Jonah's case being rejected. And if Mount Sinai says no, we have nowhere else to go. One of Dr. Wachtel's other patients gets on an airplane every week for the ECT that keeps his catatonia from recurring because he lives in a state where ECT isn't legally available for minors. But that seems so disruptive to me—not to mention costly and probably impossible given the frequency of Jonah's rages. In 2008 an autistic toddler was kicked off an American Eagle flight for "crying and screaming uncontrollably," which seems like small potatoes compared to the hitting, kicking, and biting I might expect from Jonah. The thought of just driving him two hours to New York makes me anxious enough. So I don't urge Dr. Kellner to hurry or remind him of his January prediction. I sign every email, "Thanks, Amy."

While we wait I read everything I can find about ECT, trying to understand why it's so controversial. It's as inflammatory a topic as abortion—except in abortion, at least both sides agree about what occurs during the procedure in question. The clashing forces in the ECT debate can't even get that far. Dr. Max Fink believes, "'except for penicillin for neurosyphilis and niacin for pellagra,' ECT for severe mental illness 'is the most effective treatment . . . developed in this century.'"[1] On the other hand, Leonard Roy Frank, one of the most vocal ECT "survivors" and anti-ECT crusaders, wrote in a 2010 letter to the FDA that "electroshock is a direct, violent assault on these hallmarks of American liberty: freedom of conscience, freedom of belief, freedom of thought, freedom of religion, freedom of speech, freedom from assault, and freedom from cruel and unusual punishment."[2]

How can one treatment spawn two such completely irreconcilable positions? As discussed earlier, there are many former ECT patients who feel they suffered significant side effects from their treatments. But patients have experienced severe, even fatal, side effects following every procedure imaginable—including medically unnecessary surgeries, such as liposuction. Yet nowhere is liposuction a criminal act as was ECT for a brief period in 1982 when the city of Berkeley, California, voted to prohibit the administration of ECT within the city limits. The law was voided forty-one days later by the Alameda County Superior Court.

The unmitigated animosity of the anti-ECT camp would make

sense to me if ECT didn't work. Clearly it would be wrong, even morally objectionable, to ask patients to risk even mild side effects for a therapy that had no possibility of alleviating their symptoms. But more than half a century of science has consistently shown that ECT does work. Most recently, the Consortium for Research in ECT (CORE) group, a collaboration of some of the biggest names in ECT research from institutes across the country, including Dr. Kellner and Dr. Fink, released two of the largest, multi-site studies to address this very issue. In 2006, the CORE group reported an impressive 87 percent rate of remission of symptoms among almost four hundred depressed subjects who had completed their acute courses of ECT.[3] In contrast, an ambitious study of the popular antidepressant Celexa that included almost three thousand patients under care at twenty-three different sites found that only 28 percent achieved remission after eight weeks of treatment.[4]

In a separate study on suicidal intent, the CORE group found that after just one week of ECT almost 40 percent of patients were no longer suicidal; by the end of the acute course, more than 80 percent of the subjects no longer wanted to kill themselves.[5] Antidepressants, on the other hand, can take four to six weeks to work, if they work at all. And some research suggests that patients on antidepressants may initially be at an increased risk of suicide, since their energy levels are likely to improve before their moods do.[6]

The CORE studies are by no means the only evidence out there. Researchers from around the world have documented ECT's efficacy in treating depression and mania.[7] And remission rates of over 80 percent have been recorded using ECT to treat urgent, life-threatening conditions such as catatonia, a motor syndrome whose symptoms include unresponsiveness, posturing, and purposeless movement, and neuroleptic malignant syndrome, a rare, but potentially fatal, reaction to antipsychotics.[8]

Studies on adolescents confirm that ECT is just as effective in this population as it is with adults. In 1997, Australian researchers Joseph Rey and Garry Walter analyzed every paper that had been published to date on ECT in minors. They found sixty articles, some of which had to be translated from the French, German, and Polish originals. When the authors combined the available data, they found overall improvement rates of 63 percent for depression, 80 percent for mania, 80 percent for catatonia, and 42 percent for schizophrenia, with not one death reported among the 396 included subjects.[9] (Schizophrenia is an illness for which ECT is typically prescribed today only for patients also suffering from affective, catatonic, or psychotic symptoms.) Although many of the reports were single cases and virtually all the older studies failed to follow current, rigorous, methodological protocols, one 1995 study did compare the outcomes of sixteen bipolar adolescents who received ECT to six at the same hospital who refused it in favor of medication alone. Not only did the ECT group show significantly lower scores on the Brief Psychiatric Rating Scale at discharge, but the medication-only group remained in the hospital more than twice as long: an average of 176 days compared to 74 days for the ECT group.[10]

Subsequent research has focused on adolescents with affective illnesses, such as depression and bipolar disorder, who have failed to respond to medication. These results, which were calculated using standardized testing instruments, are staggering. In one study, eleven out of eleven teens showed "clinically significant improvement," with 64 percent achieving full remission.[11] Another report from UCLA found that nine out of ten adolescents had at least halved their scores on the Hamilton Rating Scale for Depression following ECT, with six in full remission.[12] ECT works so well and so quickly that an article specifically examining its use in the intellectually disabled population expressed dismay that patients had been left to suffer years of "stupor, urinary and fecal incontinence, bedsores, shackling to the bed, profound weight loss, and psychotic experiences" before being given ECT, which improved each and every patient without causing any further cognitive impairment.[13] This echoes the conclusion Rey and Walter came to after examining more than fifty years of studies on ECT in adolescent patients: "If anything, the collective data suggest that ECT may be underutilized."

These statistics consume me as we wait: *80 percent, 100 percent, eleven out of eleven*. We wait through the snowiest winter in Philadelphia history: almost eighty inches fall over four big storms. The power goes out repeatedly, as high winds and heavy snows knock over trees in our thickly wooded neighborhood. Jonah hates the dark—he insists on sleeping with all the lights in his room on. I can tell immediately when I wake up in the middle of the night and every light in the house is on that Jonah has sneaked down to the kitchen again, his path blazing as if marked by iridescent breadcrumbs. We buy camping lanterns that consume dozens of D batteries to call into service during these blackouts, but still Jonah can focus on nothing else; he drags me by the hand to the light switches and instructs me over and over to "Fix the power," which despite his agitation and my frustration always makes me smile just a little. I can't help but think that 1960s antiestablishment types marching on Washington could have used such a pithy slogan.

The storms also cause school to be canceled and keep our aides from making it out. When I get tired of running Jonah's behavior program, I sit and draw for him. This is one of his favorite activities, one he'll do for hours: he directs me and I draw. He favors *Sesame Street* characters, but he'll also throw in random animals, or preferred family members or aides, present or past. He's very particular in his specifications: "Draw Ernie half-a-hand," he says. In the next picture, he'll want all of Ernie's hand and half his face; in the next, all of Ernie and half of Bert's hand, etc. If I sit with him long enough, he'll have me draw a series of pictures in which the characters shift across the page so I suspect if I put them together and riffled through them like a flip book they would come to life. By the end of January I feel chained to Jonah's desk. I have never loathed anything in my life more than I do Ernie and Bert. I touch base with Dr. Kellner who writes, "I plan to wait about two more weeks, before applying to the Ethics Committee." He writes, "Please stay in close touch."

When the kids are in school, I spend whatever free time I have reading: more studies, more books, some that support and others that denounce ECT. I'm trying to understand how a treatment with an 80 percent success rate can be conceived in any light as a "human rights violation," as it's described on ect.org. The more I read, the more it seems to me as if the two sides of the ECT debate aren't really divided over the question of whether ECT works. At first glance, it seems as if the anti-ECT camp believes that ECT doesn't help at all. But if you keep reading, you'll find claims like this one from Linda Andre: "The 1985 NIMH Consensus Conference finding that ECT's benefit lasts no more than four weeks stands uncontroverted."[14]

Similarly, from psychiatrist and author Peter Breggin: "[ECT] advocates were unable to come forth with a single study showing that

ECT had a positive effect beyond four weeks."[15] Even the study touted all over the web as proof that ECT isn't any better than "sham" or placebo ECT—in which patients are put under general anesthesia and believe they're getting ECT, but no current is administered—actually reports, "Real ECT causes a greater reduction in depression than sham ECT during the period of time the treatment is being administered, and for a short time after the end of treatment."[16] So, if you believe the ECT opponents, ECT does help, but not for very long.

And what if you believe ECT proponents? ECT helps a lot, but not for very long. Dr. Wachtel has made it clear from our first conversation that ECT is more like dialysis or insulin than it is like penicillin: the beneficial effects wear off over time. The duration differs for everyone. Dr. Sherwin Nuland, the surgeon and National Book Award–winning author, hasn't reported needing any ECT since the course he underwent forty years ago relieved his incapacitating depression. One mother I spoke with, whose identical twins required ECT to break their catatonia and depression, said her sons have had no maintenance ECT over the past seven years and their symptoms have remained at bay. Their family is featured in Chapter 6. On the other hand, I've also spoken to a mom whose teenage son developed catatonia so severe he suffered autonomic system failure and was at risk of death at the time he was admitted for ECT. The ECT successfully resolved the catatonia, but he still can't go more than a week without a treatment or the spells of unresponsiveness start to recur. Although we would love it if the acute course of ECT permanently stopped Jonah's aggression with no need for follow-up, we're prepared for ECT to be part of our lives for the foreseeable future.

And this is a legitimate concern about ECT: patients may require maintenance doses for years, maybe for the rest of their lives, and that's a commitment of time and money that some people may not be willing to make, although most health insurance plans at least partially cover ECT. If Jonah tapers down to a maintenance schedule of twice a month by the time he's twelve and continues to require ECT over the course of his life, he may very well get over 1,600 treatments if he lives to be seventy-five. This is a lot, no doubt, but it isn't completely unprecedented in the literature: one 1985 case study featured an eighty-nine-year-old woman who was given ECT 1,250 times over the course of her life, yet showed "no observable gross or histological sign of brain damage" upon autopsy.[17] Another study compared living patients who had all received over a hundred treatments to control subjects with the same psychiatric diagnoses and found "The two groups did not differ in any measure of objective or subjective cognitive functioning."[18]

Still, we wait. The two weeks Dr. Kellner specified pass; January becomes February. Jonah's agitation is so persistent he comes after us almost every day, often more than once. We don't want to make any major changes to his meds with ECT looming, but it's hard to see him so irritable so much of the time. His psychiatrist, Dr. James Hetznecker, bumps his Abilify up a milligram, his fourth medication increase in four months. It helps somewhat, but Jonah still engages in frequent aggression and self-injurious behavior, sometimes so intense he bloodies his own nose.

It seems clear that medication will never permanently stabilize Jonah's behavior, at least not these drugs. But the thought of going through a major pharmaceutical change with Jonah at home scares me to death. I had seen how they did it at KKI: over the course of ten months, Dr. Wachtel very slowly weaned Jonah off the Risperdal he was on at admission, then very slowly started him on Celexa, an antidepressant. She agreed with Dr. Hetznecker that Jonah had an underlying mood disorder that she assumed at first was depression. When the Celexa pushed Jonah into a manic state—a typical reaction when antidepressants are given to those with bipolar disorder— she stopped the Celexa, then very slowly started with lithium. When it became clear the lithium was really helping, she continued to increase the dose until Jonah flipped out again—unfortunately, while he was on an outing with us at a park outside of Baltimore. We couldn't understand why the SIB and the aggression had come flooding back so quickly until we returned to the NBU and talked to one of the nurses. She confirmed that Jonah's behaviors had spiked dramatically since the increase in his lithium and was paging Dr. Wachtel, even though it was a Sunday evening, because she didn't want to wait even one more day to go back to the lower dose. Going too far was the only way Dr. Wachtel could make sure she had maximized Jonah's benefit from the lithium.

This is a fine strategy when you're working in an extremely controlled environment, with as much staffing as required to take extensive data while ensuring the behaviors resulting from these pharmaceutical manipulations are safely managed. But I don't think anyone who's ever seen my home would describe it as even a barely controlled environment. There are far too many kids and far too many ways for Jonah to hurt himself or someone else for me to consider going through this process at home.

And let me add that this was the process Dr. Wachtel went through for just one drug. Most kids with behaviors as severe as Jonah's require a cocktail of two or more prescriptions to keep them even somewhat stable. When Jonah's aggression dropped but his SIB remained high, Dr. Wachtel added Abilify to Jonah's regimen. This helped for a while, but Dr. Wachtel thought she could do better so she weaned Jonah off the Abilify and started him on valproic acid (VPA), an anti-epileptic drug. According to Jonah's discharge report, "Unfortunately, despite an initial affective improvement, VPA then led to increased aggression with new-onset serious biting. VPA was thus discontinued." It turned out that Jonah was best regulated while on a combination of lithium and low-dose Abilify, and although Dr. Wachtel also tried adding a glutamate-modulating agent, riluzole, to stabilize him even further, he ended up being discharged on just the lithium and the Abilify.

As two weeks become four weeks with no word from Dr. Kellner, I start to seriously entertain the possibility that instead of the tedious, but non-threatening, bureaucratic red tape I had assumed we were facing, we may be up against a real obstacle to Jonah's ECT. If Dr. Kellner is unable to provide the ECT, or if it doesn't work as well as we hope it will, a serious pharmaceutical overhaul may be our only option. But without the twenty-four-hour support, the aides trained to respond to the most violent attacks, the constant recording of every single negative behavior so the results of each medication change can be objectively evaluated, I don't see how this is something we can do at home. So I make an appointment to visit a residential treatment facility (RTF) just a few miles away from us. This has been our safety net, the program I've mentally designated as the place Jonah will go when we can no longer keep him safely at home. Given the possibility that we may not get our ECT miracle, it seems like a mistake to put off exploring residential options much longer.

FEBRUARY 24, 2010

I'm not even sure what started this one—the pieces to the game "Block Buddies" are spilled across Jonah's desk, so he might have gotten frustrated trying to recreate a difficult pattern—but it doesn't matter; nothing could justify this disproportionate response. When I dash into Jonah's room after hearing his screams from down the hall, where I was examining the treasures Gretchen found in the bottom of the washing machine, I arrive in time to help Jonah's aide disentangle his fingers from our nanny, Marina's, collar. I direct him to the mat for a time-out, but Jonah can't calm himself down. In a few seconds, he is up and after me. Matty appears from wherever in the house he was working and is finally able to get Jonah down on the floor. The visible parts of Jonah, his face and hands, are covered with blood. He hits himself in the nose with such force it sounds like raw meat being slapped onto butcher block. You get used to a lot of things when you live with a child like Jonah; I'm not sure that sound is one of them.

We don't intervene when Jonah hits himself. This is for two reasons. First, he doesn't hurt himself that badly. This may seem like a ridiculous assessment to most parents; Jonah bloodies his nose, bruises his hips, and has pounded so often on so many hard surfaces (including his own body) that his hands are perpetually cracked and puffy. Yet I've seen much worse. There were kids at KKI who were so self-injurious they had to wear helmets and padded sleeves. There were kids who worked and ate and played at tables with protective mats on top, so when they slammed their faces down they wouldn't break their noses. If Jonah were that self-injurious, we would stop him. But because he isn't, it's just not worth putting the aides and ourselves at risk. Jonah is very, very strong. When he was in kindergarten, he kicked a teacher in the face and broke her nose during a tantrum. He has scratched me, bruised me, and pulled out my hair. Our goal in managing every tantrum is to minimize the amount of physical contact. This involves a lot of dodging Jonah's punches, twisting away from his grasp, turning him by the shoulders, and redirecting him to the floor—always careful not to let him see how upset we are. As with any kid, we never want to let Jonah know he's rattled us, thereby reinforcing the bad behavior.

It's exactly these kind of rages that have made his placement at an RTF feel inevitable. I visited the campus of the one near us last week and was impressed by what I saw—although admittedly I was predisposed to like it based on the glowing reports I'd heard from a friend of mine who has a son there. I just wish there were more information out there. I've Googled "best autism schools" to little avail; there is no big website, no central database of parent comments, incident reports, services provided—nothing. I've gathered from extensive research that there's a great school in New England, but that's too far away. Are there similarly excellent facilities in New Jersey, Pennsylvania, or Delaware? I don't know, and none of Jonah's various providers seem to know either. Not even the staff at KKI, who treat patients from all over the country, can name the most well-respected programs. This unnecessary layer of mystery only complicates what is already an incredibly hard decision.

My tour of the RTF was pretty brief. My guide, the administrator in charge of admissions for children, told me she wasn't authorized to show me any of the residences, and if I wanted to see the vocational classes, I needed to talk to a different administrator who handles the older students. But I did see the classrooms, with their enthusiastic instructors and kids not terribly dissimilar to Jonah. I saw the indoor pool where kids swim at least twice a week. And I did hear lots of good things about the vocational program, which was my chief area of interest. I've been spending a lot of time these days wondering what Jonah will do with his life. I'm struck time and again by the influence he has had on the people around him—one former aide is pursuing a career in autism research after working with Jonah while she was an undergraduate; another was moved to write a poem about him that she posted on her blog. Aides from KKI are still friending me on Facebook fourteen months after his discharge, just to see how he's doing. My typical children may never affect others so deeply. But that's a pretty abstract conception of Jonah's purpose in life. Of more pressing concern to me is how he will occupy his days once he is done with school, even though that won't be for another ten years, since children with disabilities are educated at taxpayer expense until the age of twenty-one. The Individuals with Disabilities Education Act (IDEA) mandates that planning for the transition to adulthood begin no later than age fourteen. At this particular RTF, the students are given plenty of time to experiment with different jobs before graduating, at which point they can participate in work programs, both on campus and in the community. I asked my guide whether any of these young men had aggressive behaviors. She told me they did and that those behaviors didn't necessarily preclude them from holding down jobs. Those prone to violent outbursts worked under the direct supervision of job coaches. It was such a relief to hear that, even if we fail to get Jonah's aggression completely under control, all may not be lost. For the first time in a long time I feel optimistic that Jonah will someday have a job—even if the job is menial, like deconstructing boxes at a box factory, working as a janitor at McDonald's, or shredding paper.

Typically when I stand as I'm standing now, watching Jonah thrash on the floor, I think about the RTF and ask myself, *Is it time?* I had always told myself that I would know when it was no longer safe to keep Jonah in our house; I thought there would be signs. And when I'm being honest I recognize that—unless I'm holding out for skywriting or a message flashed on the Jumbotron at a Phillies game—Andy breaking Jonah's arm and Jonah attacking our au pair in the span of a couple of weeks are signs that are about as clear as I'm likely to get. But that's not what I'm thinking now as Jonah sits up and takes an exaggeratedly deep breath, which his teachers have taught him to do to help calm himself down. My heart breaks when I see him try so hard to pull himself together because so many of these attempts end up as this one does: with Jonah sprawled on his back once again, kicking and crying, with no more than ten or fifteen seconds elapsed on the stopwatch we use to clock his one-minute time-outs. This means we have to stop the timer, re-set it to one minute, and wait for him to sit calmly before we start it again. Matty remains in the room, leaning against the edge of Jonah's desk; his aide, Candace, controls the stopwatch. Usually by the time Jonah drops to the floor he's no longer aggressive, but Matty just wants to be sure.

No, I'm not thinking about the RTF as Jonah sits up again, as he tells Candace, "Yes," the code for "I'm ready, start the timer, now I'm calm." This time, I'm thinking about the email from Dr. Kellner I received just a few hours ago: "Hold-up is over." He is ready to present Jonah's case to the ethics committee. Hopefully, I won't have to fight with my son very much longer.

MARCH 2, 2010

Dr. Kellner doesn't keep me in suspense. The subject line in his email says it all: "Ethics Committee Approves." In the body of his email he notes how helpful the pictures I sent him of Jonah bloodying his own nose (not last week's episode, but one dating several months back) were in swaying the Committee. This makes me smile. It's amazing how useful those pictures have been in getting the attention of administrators and government officials. It also reminds me, as so much does, of the enormous gulf between my friends and me. What kind of parent runs and gets a camera while her son is punching himself in the face? I did. And when Jonah wasn't getting the number of hours of support for which he was authorized by the state insurance company, I sent out those pictures to everyone I could think of: the insurance company, the Secretary of Public Welfare, the Deputy Secretary for Mental Health and Substance Abuse Services. I heard from the insurance company the day my letter was received, a meeting was immediately scheduled, and ever since then I get periodic phone calls from Jonah's care manager to see how things are going. I guess a picture really is worth ten thousand angry, beseeching, threatening words.

Dr. Kellner and I talk on the phone later. There are two tests Jonah needs before we can start ECT: a baseline MRI and a test for a very rare genetic condition, Lesch-Nyhan Syndrome. This disease causes mental retardation and self-injurious behavior (primarily biting) but also causes kidney problems, which Jonah has never had. The genetic test is easy—well, easy for me, since it will have to be Andy who holds Jonah down while his blood is drawn. But the MRI will require anesthesia, since there's no way Jonah will lie still for forty-five minutes while a machine images his brain.

Fortunately, I already have an appointment scheduled with Dr. Hetznecker for the next morning. I hope he will be able to order these tests, and we can get them done immediately. Dr. Kellner tells me that, optimally, Jonah could get his first ECT in about ten days.

CHAPTER 4

Paul

In January 1993, Teri underwent amniocentesis to check her four-month-old fetus for genetic defects. Her three-year-old daughter, Amanda, had been born with tuberous sclerosis (TSC), which causes the growth of benign tumors on the brain, heart, kidneys, and other organs. Up to 60 percent of those with this disorder suffer from intellectual disability; co-diagnoses of autism, ADHD, OCD, and mood disorders are common. Although Amanda seemed to be developing typically, she did suffer from seizures—as do up to 90 percent of individuals with TSC. She was also at risk for polycystic kidney disease and lymphangioleiomyomatosis, a degenerative lung disease, as she grew into adulthood. Given the uncertain prognosis of kids with TSC, Teri and her husband, Steve, had decided to terminate the pregnancy if their fetus had a major defect.

Teri didn't know that her practice had only recently begun offering amniocentesis, so her doctor was inexperienced with the procedure. But she vividly remembered how his hands shook as he slid the needle into her belly. And she won't ever forget how the point struck her baby's skull, how it drew a thin plume of blood. The doctor didn't say anything, and Teri and Steve were too consumed with the possibility that their unborn child might have a major disability to worry about something that didn't concern the OB/GYN. When the genetic tests came back negative, Teri and Steve finally allowed themselves to celebrate the impending arrival of their healthy son.

But it wasn't long after Paul's birth before it became clear there was something wrong. He had trouble turning his head to nurse and was diagnosed with "failure to thrive." It wasn't until Paul was still unable to hold up his head at four months that Teri and Steve discovered exactly why: an MRI revealed that Paul had suffered an in utero stroke. As a result he had been born with only half a cerebellum, the part of the brain that controls balance and coordination, and contributes as well to language and attention. Although his doctors had never seen a case like Paul's, they were optimistic. They speculated that his biggest problems would be with gross motor development. They told Teri and Steve, "He'll never be an Olympic athlete."

———

Paul, who was sixteen when I met him at his home in January 2010, is not an Olympic athlete. He's not even verbal. My first impression was of a profoundly impaired young man: his asymmetrical brain causes him to perpetually tilt his head to the right; he lurches when he walks; he grunts when he's excited. It's understandable, I suppose, why his teachers and school administrators assumed that Paul was incapable of learning or communicating. What's not so understandable is why they refused to reconsider their first impressions when Teri repeatedly told them that Paul had a sign language vocabulary several hundred signs strong, that he just needed modified instructional materials, that he threw tantrums out of frustration with not being able to articulate his needs.

Instead, Paul was placed in a typical kindergarten class at his public school with a teacher who refused to learn sign language. Because Paul couldn't write yet, he had no way to communicate with her. By first grade, he was given a Dynavox 2C, a big, heavy, assisted-communication device. But, Teri told me, its vocabulary was "extremely limited—yes, no, I'm thirsty, I need to go to the bathroom." Teri lobbied for a more functional device for her son, but was told he had neither the fine motor skills nor the cognitive abilities to use it. His outbursts—during which Paul would bite, hit, and scratch both his teachers and his classmates—were due, the teachers informed Teri, to her lack of discipline. It took another four years of pleading before the school district relented and provided a replacement device to Paul when he was eleven. The same night he brought the Vantage with an updated Picture Wordpower program home, Paul figured out the system of picture, word, and letter keys and started "talking" in complete sentences.

It was amazing for me to converse with Paul and his Vantage. Unlike the controversial and now discredited technique of facilitated communication, in which severely low-functioning autistics are physically prompted by "facilitators" to tap out messages on a keyboard, Paul (who is not autistic) does all his own typing. As any other kid would do, he bugged his mom for help, and as any other mom would do, Teri encouraged Paul to do it himself. "You know how to spell that," she said when he held up the Vantage to show her what he was writing. We chatted about the bird feeder we could see through the sliding glass doors that led out to the deck. If anything slowed Paul down, it was his insistence on typing out complete sentences, including my name, which Teri did help him spell. "Santa Claus brought me a bird osprey book for Christmas, Amy," he told me. On the cold winter day of my visit, we saw no ospreys, nor did we see any pelicans, which Paul told me were his favorite birds. "We saw pelicans down in Florida," the Vantage said in its robotic voice.

Although the assisted communication device was a huge success in enabling Paul to interact with the world, it didn't do much to reduce his aggressive behavior. By the age of twelve, his rages had grown so intense he would throw furniture across the room until one of his parents restrained him in a basket hold on the floor. During his worst fits, he slammed his head through the windows. The staff at Paul's school, aside from suspending Paul for biting the principal, had no counsel to offer them. The teachers continued to blame Teri for spoiling him; the school district threatened to send him to a school for emotionally disturbed kids unless he was medicated. A psychiatrist recommended Risperdal, which did help. "It actually seemed like a miracle," Teri said. "It reduced his anger to a point that we could actually implement some behavior programs, which then worked." But about a year later, Paul started developing tics—a common side effect of Risperdal—so Teri and Steve stopped it immediately. Happily, Paul's behavior remained relatively stable through fifth grade. His parents allowed themselves to hope their son would never again need antipsychotics.

When Paul graduated from elementary school, the district announced its intention to place him in a catch-all Special Ed class with thirteen other students with various disabilities, one teacher, and very little support. Teri knew Paul would never thrive in this situation, so she decided to home-school him.

"I actually loved homeschooling," she said—which, I confess, did not reflect my own experience. I homeschooled Jonah for four months while we waited for a bed to open up at KKI, and even though our district provided a teacher who came to the house for a few hours every morning, I found the whole experience completely draining.

Teri, in contrast, didn't have any help at all. "It was the best academic environment he ever had, and he learned the most that year and a half. We had a great routine, where he would wake up very anxious to run down to the basement that we had set up like a classroom. I would put our 'agenda' on the dry erase board and we would spend several hours each morning working. The first thing he did was a journal entry. That was followed by a game, some math, some spelling. some writing, and reading." She laughed. "He loved learning about the old days."

But caring for Paul all day, every day, took its toll. By February 2007 Teri was exhausted. "I ended up with a serious migraine problem which left me fairly debilitated," she admitted. Fortunately, since the time that Teri had pulled Paul from the public school, a new principal had been hired who adapted the classroom Teri had initially rejected, providing new equipment and additional staff. Teri and Steve approved the new environment, and Paul returned to school. They also decided to try Risperdal again. Although they were still concerned about its side effects, they had to do something about Paul's escalating rages, which had been difficult enough to manage when he was younger. At thirteen, he was almost as big as Teri.

This time around, however, the Risperdal only helped for a few months. Paul's behavior worsened to the point where he would attack his father, his sister—anyone who was near him. Teri and Steve stopped taking him out in the community because they were too afraid he might hurt someone. Paul was especially, inexplicably, provoked by babies and would lunge after infants wherever he saw them.

"At some point I knew we wouldn't be able to manage," Teri said when I asked if they ever considered a residential placement. "But we didn't know what we were going to do." No one, it seemed, had any answers for her. Paul's school refused to spend money on additional services; consulting sessions with local experts proved fruitless. Teri and Steve felt completely isolated. Even Teri's extensive family could no longer help, as Paul grew bigger and his tantrums worsened. If Teri had to run to the store or do some other urgent errand, the only one she could leave Paul with aside from Steve—who was often working—was her daughter, Amanda, who had been taught the basket hold restraint technique when she was only thirteen years old.

Paul's rage peaked when he was fourteen in February 2008. In consultation with Paul's doctors, Teri weaned him off the Risperdal and tried different medications to control his aggression, but those either failed to help or made him worse. Then in March, Paul had his first catatonic episode, although his parents had no idea what it was at the time.

"He went into a stupor that lasted eight days," Teri told me. "He couldn't feed himself or go to school. He lost continence. He would spend hours frozen, lying with his head lifted inches off the ground." This position, called psychological pillow, is a classic catatonic posture, but Paul's neurologist happened to be in Australia and was unable to diagnose it from the email descriptions Teri sent. Paul's developmental pediatrician thought he might be having seizures, but his EEG was normal, so Teri and Paul were sent to the Emergency Room to check for hydrocephalus. It was just one of three trips Paul made to the ER by the end of March, for symptoms as bizarre as lip smacking, eye blinking, profuse sweating, temperature irregulation, insomnia alternating with excessive sleeping, and head and stomach pain. And the worst symptom: Paul stopped using his Vantage. He wouldn't communicate with Teri and Steve at all.

But it wasn't hydrocephalus, either. Once that was ruled out, the developmental pediatrician asked her receptionist to inform Teri that her son was no longer welcome in the practice. Support from their families and friends dwindled to an all-time low, since there didn't seem to be any medical reason for Paul's behavior. Without answers once again, all Teri and Steve could do was watch as Paul cycled: eight to ten days of total unresponsiveness, followed by the same period of raging. In total, Paul had three episodes of catatonia before his neurologist, back in the United States, reached a child psychiatrist at Johns Hopkins who immediately recognized the catatonic symptoms and put Teri and Steve in touch with Dr. Wachtel.

At first, Teri and Steve wanted to try controlling Paul's catatonia with medication; Dr. Wachtel recommended first-line anticatatonic treatment with lorazepam. The benzodiazepine snapped the stupor immediately, but did little to alleviate Paul's tantrums; that summer, he kicked out the windshield of a car. He still couldn't use the Vantage and missed almost three months of school. When he did return, he often didn't last the whole day. "He would get stuck at the computer and his teacher would call me to come get him," Teri said, re-calling how she would find Paul hunched over the keyboard, pushing the same button over and over. "It would take three or four people to carry him screaming out to the car."

When the lorazepam wasn't enough, lithium and Paxil were added to Paul's regimen. This cocktail seemed to help, but the doses had to be constantly increased until Dr. Wachtel was afraid to push any higher because of the risk of side effects, including dangerous imbal-ance that caused Paul to fall and put his hand through a glass door, requiring stitches. Then, in January, Teri took Paul and Amanda to the Smithsonian where he had what Teri describes as a "psychotic meltdown."

"He was very aggressive, out of control," she remembered. "Amanda and I had to use a two-man carry to get him out of the mu-seum. The police came—it was horrible. It took Paul at least an hour outside to calm down." It was after this that Teri and Steve agreed to ECT, which Dr. Wachtel had originally presented as an alternative if the medications ever stopped working.

Amanda, back in college after her Christmas break, was devas-tated when she heard the news. Prescribed Tegretol since childhood to control the seizures caused by TSC, it seemed crazy to her to inten-tionally induce seizures in her brother's brain. Even more ominous was the realization that her parents' decision meant they had run out of options. Concerned about possible side effects from both the general anesthesia and the muscle relaxant used in the procedure—although, interestingly, not from the ECT itself—Teri and Steve had initially resisted ECT. Their reversal revealed to Amanda just how desperate the situation was.

It was easy to talk about all this a year later, with Paul sitting calmly on the floor by his mother's chair, listening—and, occasion-ally, contributing—to the conversation, which lasted several hours. Watching him, I found it hard to imagine this attentive teen attack-ing his grandmother, shattering the glass in his shower stall, or de-stroying, as Teri told me, "every piece of furniture in the house." But I could say the same thing about every child I've met with this degree of aggressive behavior, including Jonah: until you have witnessed that Jekyll-and-Hyde transformation first-hand, until you've seen a child explode into an unreachable, irrational, cyclone of fury, so foreign, yet so familiar—well, it is impossible to believe. Sometimes, it's impossible to believe even after you've seen it.

I asked Paul if he liked to go to ECT, and he typed on the Vantage, tugging on Teri's arm again to help him with my name: "I feel better after ECT, Amy."

It was the Vantage that illustrated the dramatic impact ECT had on Paul; after just one treatment he began using it again, following months of being unable to express his thoughts. Four treatments later, both the catatonia and the alternating rage were gone. And neither has returned. Paul was on a maintenance schedule of one treatment every two weeks, which seems to be the longest any of the adolescents I've met can go without their catatonic, aggressive, and/ or self-injurious symptoms returning. It's not cheap—at $325 a pop *after* insurance, Paul's ECT was a tremendous strain on the family's finances. All that mattered to Teri and Steve, however, was that Paul was back to his favorite activities: hiking, skiing, boating, and—just like his mother who still competed—swimming. Sometimes Steve took Paul to Teri's swim meets to cheer her on.

"He's not perfect," Teri said. "Sometimes, he still gets 'stuck,' and if Steve or I decide we need to make him move on, we may have to carry him, and he may yell and resist. But no biting, no scratching, no breaking anything." In fact, Paul's behavior was so stable that Teri and Steve were able to take both their kids to Florida in the fall of 2009. It was their first trip in over two-and-a-half years.

"Did you see any alligators in Florida?" I asked Paul.

"I didn't see any alligators in Florida," he told me. "I saw an iguana, Amy." And Teri found a picture in the kitchen: a photograph of Paul, kneeling in the middle of a road with a huge grin on his face, pointing at the enormous lizard they had found just crossing the street, as unremarkable there as a squirrel or chipmunk would be in their own neighborhood.

During my visit, we discussed the potential side effects of the ECT that Paul would likely require for the rest of his life. Teri and Steve hadn't noticed any cognitive deterioration or memory loss, but they had scheduled neuropsychological testing for Paul to make sure. In 2012 Dr. Wachtel would publish the results in the journal *Pediatric Neurology*: after sixty-one treatments, Paul's Nonverbal Intelligence Quotient was actually slightly *higher* than it had been during an assessment five years earlier, before ECT. This led Dr. Wachtel and her co-authors to conclude, "These findings support the lack of deleterious cognitive effects after acute and maintenance electroconvulsive therapy in pediatric and neurodevelopmentally disabled patients."

Even with those findings pending, it was obvious when I met him how drastically ECT had improved the quality of life of Paul and his family. He showed me essays he typed for school on his Vantage about the American Revolution and about his plans for the future. He was inspired primarily by the janitors he loved at his old school, though Teri suspected his future will involve a job like data entry that requires less gross motor planning. Paul's ability to articulate his thoughts was so impressive that I couldn't help but ask him what I always wanted to ask Jonah, what I did sometimes ask out of sheer frustration, knowing even as the words flew from my lips he would never be able to answer: "Why did you used to get so mad?"

Paul typed furiously. "I always get mad because I want to watch *Harry Potter and the Chamber of Secrets* on TV," the Vantage announced momentarily.

Teri laughed. "Maybe that used to cause a tantrum," she said. "But no longer."

CHAPTER 5

Jonah, march 2010

ECT BEGINS

MARCH 16, 2010

Andy and I pick Jonah up at school at eleven for the two-hour-plus drive to New York. Jonah's first ECT isn't scheduled until tomorrow morning, but first he has to meet with a child psychiatrist at Mount Sinai, Dr. Alex Kolevzon, to satisfy New York State requirements that, in cases involving children aged thirteen or younger, two consultants, "at least one being independent, who are experienced in the treatment of children," agree that ECT is indicated. I'm assuming this is just routine—like the MRI and the genetic test, both of which came back negative—a kind of rubber-stamping. Still, I'm a little anxious. Dr. Kolevzon has scheduled an hour and a half to meet with us. That seems like a long time for a rubber stamp.

We take the Lincoln Tunnel and drive crosstown, then up to the Mount Sinai campus at 99th and Madison. As we sit in the always impenetrable New York traffic I imagine doing this without Andy, as I suspect I will be doing most days. It just doesn't make sense for Andy to take so much time off work. As tough as it will be to get Jonah in the car by five o'clock and drive two hours, during which he can neither drink nor eat—though I have no doubt he'll be asking the whole time—the fact is the ECT team at Mount Sinai is well staffed and prepared for all the intricacies of treating a kid like Jonah, even though they haven't treated many children there at all. Liz Muller, the ECT nurse, told me there have been just two since Dr. Kellner arrived last year. Still, she understands that Jonah will have to be held down for his IV to be inserted, that he will wake up agitated, and that he will want to leave as soon as he can stand. She is ready to handle all these contingencies: she tells me they have several strong orderlies who can help restrain Jonah for the IV, at which point his sedative will be administered immediately; she will be ready with a dose of Versed to calm him down if he wakes up agitated. In fact, we will be able to leave without delay. So we won't necessarily require Andy's muscle, as we so often do during medical procedures. As much as I would love him to be there, especially on the long drives when I'll be tired and anxious about possible behaviors from my exhausted, bored, hungry, thirsty son, I know I can do this by myself.

We get to Dr. Kolevzon's office just in time for our two o'clock appointment. I'm not sure what I was expecting: definitely a Russian accent, probably someone slight, bearded, and older—kind of like Dr. Kellner. But Dr. Kolevzon is young and tall with Patrick Dempsey hair. In his completely accentless voice, he asks Andy to take Jonah for a walk for forty-five minutes so he and I can talk about Jonah.

Every new doctor, therapist, administrator always asks the same questions. It used to drive me bonkers, the sheer repetitiveness of it all. Were there any complications in my pregnancy or delivery? Did Jonah meet his milestones on time? Is there other mental illness in my family? Really basic questions one would think a new provider could find the answers to by taking a minute to flip through Jonah's records. Jonah must have a paper trail a mile long—I'm sure Dr. Kolevzon, for example, received some kind of assessment from Dr. Kellner who, I would also imagine, has been in contact with Dr. Wachtel. But I've come to hope that perhaps there's some kind of reason for all this repetition. Maybe, just maybe, one day I'll remember something I never mentioned before, something that might cause a light bulb to go on in the new doctor's head. If not to me, maybe it happens to another mom describing to yet another provider how her disabled child was the product of a completely uneventful, vaginal birth. John and Cheryl, Greg's parents, compiled a dossier they hand to every new practitioner. It details every notable event in their son's life: every doctor, every hospital, every medication. But somehow I suspect they're still asked the same questions over and over. In the world of autism, these questions have become a sort of catechism, a ritual used to establish a relationship between parent and doctor.

After Dr. Kolevzon and I have engaged in this particular dance long enough, I ask him some questions. Has he treated many kids like Jonah? As the Clinical Director of the Seaver Autism Center for Research and Treatment at Mount Sinai School of Medicine, he has.

I know from what he has told me that he doesn't have much experience with ECT, so I ask what has worked with his patients. He tells me that generally a cocktail of meds is required and that he keeps trying different combinations until something works. He suggests that Clozaril might be helpful for Jonah, although he admits it's an intense drug, with a side effect profile that requires blood testing every two weeks. I don't even ask what the side effects are. The possibility of getting Jonah off high-octane antipsychotics is one of the main reasons we're doing ECT in the first place, and I'm just not ready to think about what will happen if it doesn't work.

So I don't really respond to Dr. Kolevzon's suggestion that I consider Clozaril. Instead, I ask him whether his patients like Jonah are still living at home when they're twelve, thirteen, fourteen. "Only those who can't find appropriate residential placements," he tells me. Puberty will likely make Jonah worse, he continues. His aggression and his self-injurious behaviors will just get more intense.

I must look stunned because Dr. Kolevzon adds that a residential placement now doesn't have to be forever. "These kids come out on the other side of puberty with more impulse control," he tells me. "They do develop—maybe not typically, but they do mature." He says that he can tell, just from the few seconds that he's observed Jonah so far, that Jonah isn't severely retarded and guesses that his IQ is close to normal (meaning seventy or above). That fact—combined with Jonah's abilities to read, write and talk—are all signs of a good prognosis. But for now Dr. Kolevzon suggests that perhaps my goal to keep Jonah at home isn't the right one—not for Jonah and not for us. He is concerned about everyone's safety, but it's more than that. He points out that we cannot possibly duplicate in our chaotic household the level of structure offered by a residential facility—structure that, based on his success at KKI, Jonah seems to thrive on.

"We have a lot of help," I tell him. "There's almost always an aide with Jonah when he gets home from school and on most weekends."

"Don't you think Jonah would enjoy being surrounded by people who understand him and other kids who are like him?" he asks.

"I'm not sure Jonah understands that he's not like other kids," I say, although the truth is, I have no idea what Jonah understands or doesn't understand. The autism world is filled with amazing stories, such as that of Tito Mukhopadhyay, a profoundly autistic and non-verbal young man from India, whose mother famously taught him to communicate so well that at the age of eleven his poetry and essays drew international attention. But Jonah already knows how to write; in fact, he could write before he could talk. I'm not sure how old he was when he taught himself, but we found out when he was four and started writing in chalk on the driveway. It was mostly *Sesame Street* video titles at the beginning: *The Best of Ernie and Bert*, or *Big Bird Sings*. Once, he wrote "FBI Warning," which inspired from Andy a bastardized quote from *The Princess Bride*: "Jonah, I don't think those words mean what you think they mean." Now . . . it's still a lot of *Sesame Street* titles. No poetry. No philosophy. One summer afternoon, Jonah did write something that caused my hope to skyrocket (and made me run for my camera to capture the words before the next rainstorm washed them away): "EACH DAY I LIKE IT BETTER." This didn't sound at all familiar to me, as his other scripted phrases did—could it possibly be an original statement, one reflecting a new self-awareness, an optimistic embrace of the future? That's what I believed until Keri Googled the line and found it was, in fact, part of a *Sesame Street* song called "Dee, Dee, Dee": "'D' is such a very nice letter. Each day I like it better, that lovely letter called 'D!'" I continued to draw consolation from the fact that Jonah must have had some reason for picking that particular line (rather than, say, "Don't drop dishes down on the floor"); we still have no real evidence, however, of whether he ever thinks about anything more profound than what he says to us, such as the request he makes virtually every morning before he gets on the van to go to school: "Mommy, I want drive to water park, roller coaster park, beach, Sesame Place, swimming, mall, ketchup and French fries, cinnamon sugar pretzel in Mr. Boss's [his teacher's] car. Please."

I always say, "If it's okay with Mr. Boss, it's okay with me."

I always think, *If I could peek inside the mind of anyone in the entire world, it would be yours, Jonah.*

Dr. Kolevzon says, "That kind of insight comes with age."

I pause, considering what has transpired. Dr. Kolevzon has just done what none of Jonah's doctors ever had before: he said that Jonah would likely be better off in a residential placement. Slowly, the magnitude of this moment settles through me. I, like many parents forced to consider removing their children from their own homes, have struggled to decipher my own opaque motivations. No doubt, my life would be easier if Jonah were in an RTF. Andy and I could take our four other kids and get on a plane and spend Christmas break somewhere warm, just as I long to do every year. Never mind vacations—we could take the kids bike riding, or bowling, or to the dog park. We wouldn't have to split the family up every weekend, with Andy taking Jonah to BJ's or on a hike while I take the other kids to soccer games, movies, or birthday parties. We could relax at home without being afraid that whenever our attention was diverted, Jonah would gorge in the kitchen, write on the walls, or sneak outside through a door accidentally pulled only partially shut. Most importantly, we could stop worrying that Jonah would seriously hurt one of his siblings or cousins, or one of their little friends. Because, honestly—if, God forbid, that should happen, who could say we shouldn't have seen it coming?

Given all these factors, it surprises me that Dr. Kolevzon's permission doesn't give me anything resembling a sense of freedom. Rather, it fills me with despair. My family will still be divided, I realize—and no matter what hopeful predictions Dr. Kolevzon makes about the future, it may very well be forever. "I just don't want to give up too early," I say, thinking about ECT and the possibility that we may be permanently rid of these aggressive behaviors. Why not? Teri, Paul's mother, told me that her son hasn't had one aggressive tantrum since he started ECT. It could be the same for Jonah. Even if the two boys Dr. Kolevzon has seen treated with ECT have only shown "modest" improvements, that hasn't been Dr. Wachtel's experience. Eleven out of eleven, I remind myself. This has become my mantra.

"You're not giving up," Dr. Kolevzon says. "And it's not too early."

Andy knocks on the door, back from his walk with Jonah. Dr. Kolevzon asks if he can do a brief assessment of Jonah, who is literally bouncing off the walls of his office, like usual.

"Jonah, what day is it?" Dr. Kolevzon asks.

Given how agitated Jonah seems, confined to Dr. Kolevzon's tiny office, I think we're all surprised when Jonah says, "Tuesday."

"That's right, Jonah. And what year is it?" Dr. Kolevzon asks.

"Wednesday," Jonah mutters. This is a pattern of his—when you start asking him questions, he tries to anticipate what the next question will be and guess the information you're trying to elicit from him without actually processing the question.

"Do you know what season it is, Jonah?" Dr. Kolevzon tries.

Andy and I find ourselves repeating the questions, sure that Jonah will pay more attention to us, his parents, then this complete stranger. Eventually, Jonah offers, "Fall."

"Not quite," Andy says.

"Winter," Jonah says.

There's a pause, because the weather is beautiful outside, sunny and warm. But spring is officially still four days away. "Yes, it is winter," Andy says.

While he's observing Jonah, Dr. Kolevzon gives me two surveys to fill out cataloging Jonah's behaviors. He says that we will do these assessments again in about six weeks to determine if the ECT has had any effect. Jonah, meanwhile, is getting more and more agitated. He doesn't actually come after any of us, but he does end up on the floor, screaming and thrashing around.

"And there's nothing you can say when he gets like this?" Dr. Kolevzon asks. "You just have to wait?"

That's what we do, we wait. Dr. Kolevzon looks over the papers I've completed and notes, "Aggression is a severe problem . . . and his pacing and spinning are also pretty severe. These other things—the list making, the object arranging—we're not going to worry about those for now."

After we leave Mount Sinai, Andy, Jonah, and I head to Andy's best friend Adam's apartment in midtown. The New York office of Andy's firm is only a few blocks from there, and we are meeting Jen—a former long-time aide of Jonah's who is now working as a receptionist at said office—for dinner. After a brief moment of confusion during which Andy discovers that Adam is in San Diego, despite the fact that he told Andy we could stay over, the doorman lets us in and we drop off our stuff. We then head over to Outback: a great compromise restaurant for our family, since it serves French fries, Jonah's favorite, but the food doesn't come wrapped in cardboard and wax paper.

It's great to see Jen. Although she majored in English and is currently waiting to hear from several graduate programs, she was an amazing aide and Jonah really loves her. She worked with him after school, at sleep-away camp, and at our shore house. She fills us in on her life while we wait for our food. Jonah is very patient, even while we eat our salads. He watches his iTouch and participates a little in the conversation, eyeing every waiter who walks by in the hopes he's bearing his hamburger and French fries. Jonah is very well behaved in restaurants—much better than the twins—and can wait forever as long as he knows French fries are coming. Once he is done eating, however, he wants to leave. Immediately. Fortunately, we finish only about thirty seconds after Jonah decides the only way to escape our booth is to slip to the floor and slide under the bench. We head out for a walk through Central Park.

It's a lovely evening. After the longest, coldest, snowiest winter on record, it feels divine just to stroll outside as the sun sets. Andy and Jonah climb a gigantic rock, while Jen and I relax on a bench beneath. I describe my conversation with Dr. Kolevzon and tell her that in the car on our way downtown, Andy had commented, "You seem sad." When I asked him why he wasn't sad to hear Dr. Kolevzon's recommendation, he shrugged. "I just want to do what's best for Jonah. If a residential placement is better for him, then that's what we'll do." It seems so screwed-up, such a through-the-looking-glass kind of world, where it's better for children to be separated from their parents. But the autism world is very different from the typical world. I wonder when that will stop surprising me.

Jen doesn't really know what to say. What is there to say, really? But it's nice to sit with her. And Jonah has a great evening. He absolutely loves New York—a place I thought would give him sensory overload. But he doesn't seem to care about the noise or the crowds. There's a soft pretzel vendor on every corner and that makes the city paradise to him. The entire walk back from the park, he tries everything he can think of to get us to leave him alone, to go to some hypothetical bathroom, to walk into a store—to do anything, in other words, that would free him to prowl the streets of New York, eating himself sick on soft pretzels. And I have no doubt he would score many. Last summer, while we were all at one of the amusement piers in Ocean City, Jonah got away from us while Andy and I were swapping roles: he was going to take Jonah to the water park a few blocks down, and I was going to take Erika and Hilary on rides. (Our nanny was assigned to chaperone the twins, since all Aaron ever wanted to do was ride the carousel over and over and over again; one of the tremendous advantages of having a nanny is being able to delegate these types of tasks). We split up to look for Jonah. I headed right toward the beach—Jonah loves the ocean and that seemed to me the biggest threat to his safety. (I don't worry too much about abduction; I almost pity the pedophile that tries to kidnap Jonah). Plus, I figured that one of the lifeguards would be able to send out the alert by walkie-talkie if I didn't immediately find him—which I did. He was strolling along the water's edge, his shoes gone, a churro in his hand. I immediately threw the churro in a trash can because I didn't want to reward his running away from us, but I was secretly impressed by his industriousness; he had, after all, only been gone for a few minutes. I couldn't stop wondering how he got the churro. Did he snatch it out of someone's hand? Or maybe he just walked up to a stand, said, "Churro," and was handed one by someone who expected payment?

Although Jonah is tired after our pretzel-free walk back to Adam's apartment, it takes him a long time to fall asleep. Following Dr. Kellner's instructions, I don't give Jonah his lithium or his melatonin in preparation for tomorrow's ECT. I know at least the melatonin, a natural supplement you can buy in any drug or vitamin store, really helps him sleep. When it's after ten and Jonah still keeps getting out of bed, I tell Andy that it's silly for both of us to wait him out. I go in to Jonah's room and snuggle with him, something I do many nights. It's such a peaceful way to wrap up the day and he always asks so sweetly, "Mommy, lie down," that I rarely say no. No matter what may have transpired earlier—whether Jonah hit me, scratched me, or yanked my favorite necklace right off my neck—it's nice to settle into the quiet and feel, as I rarely do with my other children, the sheer physical weight of the love that remains once the frustration, the grief, and the fear dissolve like bad dreams into the night. Even after the worst of days, I can watch sleep smooth the pain from Jonah's beautiful face and believe, really believe, each and every time, that tomorrow will be better.

Jonah's asleep by eleven thirty, but I bounce in and out of sleep all night. I'm not sure if it's anxiety about the upcoming ECT that keeps me awake, excitement about ECT, or just sharing a bed with Jonah, who wedges himself against me, following me unconsciously even if I try to create some space between us. I could go back and sleep with Andy, but I'm afraid that Jonah might wake up and slip out of Adam's apartment without us hearing. Our doors at home are fitted with combination locks so no one can get in or out without pushing the right sequence of buttons. This is a solution we arrived at several years ago when Jonah went through an escape phase. We tried every childproof device on the market with no success; he would solve, in about thirty seconds, complicated gadgets my in-laws were utterly unable to manipulate. Fortunately, the escape phase coincided with a naked phase. Motorists might just shake their heads at a seven-year-old walking along the side of our busy road, but they reliably called 911 to report a seven-year-old walking along the side of our busy road in his underwear. It took two visits from the police department before we managed—through the combination locks, plus assorted key locks—to seal off every possible means of egress, including a bathroom window six feet off the ground and a warped and forgotten basement door. I still can't help but marvel, sometimes, at the basic bolts on my friends' doors: shiny and simple and in easy reach of little hands, yet their kids never just . . . leave.

Jonah likes to tuck my palm under his cheek when he goes to sleep. He always asks for "Mommy's right hand," even though it's the left hand he wants; it's just that, when he looks at me, my preferred hand is on *his* right. I've tried explaining, but this is one of those things he just doesn't get. A lack of empathy, of being able to see things from another person's perspective, is a textbook autistic trait. Because I'm a mother who firmly believes in picking her battles—and because of all Jonah's battles, this one clearly isn't worth fighting—I don't correct him anymore. Instead, when he murmurs in his sleep, "Mommy's right hand," groping across the blanket until he finds it, I let him pull my left hand to him and slide it beneath his face. I always wonder if he thinks this light pressure is enough to keep me trapped beside him, if he does this because he doesn't want me to get up once he falls asleep. Tonight this plan will work.

MARCH 17, 2010

Staying overnight in New York definitely makes the ECT logistics easier. We wake Jonah up, throw some clothes on, jump in the car, and we're at Mount Sinai ten minutes later, just after seven.

There's not enough time for Jonah to realize he has neither eaten breakfast nor had anything to drink. On Wednesday, when I drive Jonah up to Mount Sinai by myself from home, I anticipate that his hunger and especially his thirst will be real problems.

We check in at the registration area. After about half an hour, during which I grow increasingly impatient, an orderly appears to walk us up to the post-anesthesia care unit (PACU) that is co-opted by the ECT team during these early morning hours. We're greeted by Dr. Kellner and his nurse, Liz, who in short order introduce us to the anesthesiologist and various other medical personnel I have trouble keeping track of. Despite the fact that not many children are treated by the ECT team, they understand how imperative it is that Jonah be in and out as quickly as possible—unless they want to witness the type of tantrum Jonah threw in Dr. Kolevzon's office. Within a few minutes after our approval by the anesthesiologist, Jonah is being held down on the gurney by five people—including two doctors, a nurse, an orderly, and Andy—to have his IV inserted. As Jonah struggles against the restraint, we all hear a loud pop, like cracking knuckles, but louder. Andy jumps, releasing Jonah's arm. "Oh, my God," he says. "I didn't hurt him again, did I?"

The doctors pause to check Jonah who is, in fact, holding his arm against his chest, as he did after it was broken. But the doctors and nurses all agree that the sound didn't sound like a bone breaking, but just a joint cracking. They promise to do a more thorough examination when he's sedated. They take their places around him a second time—all except Andy, who can't bring himself to lay hands on Jonah again—and within a few seconds, the IV is in, the drugs are injected, and Jonah is asleep. The team wheels Jonah's bed to the ECT machine in the corner and pulls the drapes. We're told to take a walk, to go get some coffee. Family members aren't permitted to watch the actual procedure for the same reason they're not permitted to observe surgeries: some might find even the slight physical manifestations of the seizure upsetting (based on the YouTube video I found these may include clenched toes and rapid breathing). Doctors also want to spare parents in the extremely unlikely event that something goes wrong and emergency measures are required. Andy and I aren't particularly concerned. The death rate from ECT is about 1 in 10,000, no greater than that of general anesthesia alone, making it one of the safest procedures for which general anesthesia is indicated. And Jonah's been under twice before: once, to have his tonsils and adenoids removed, and once to repair a chipped tooth, so we know he tolerates it well. What we are is starving.

Although the seizure only takes between two and three minutes, the anesthesia takes a while to wear off. Liz promises to sit with Jonah if he stirs before we get back, so Andy and I head down to the cafeteria to grab something to eat. We're also on the lookout for a soft pretzel, which was prominently featured on the list Andy and Jonah had typed out on Andy's iPhone while we were waiting in the registration area. We often make lists to structure Jonah's time. He loves doing it and it really seems to help calm him. This past Christmas break, for example, Andy and I took the kids to Hershey Park, and Jonah was having trouble waiting for the soft pretzel that had been promised him. He was agitated and crying when Andy got the brilliant idea to type a list using the note app on his iPhone:

1. Gliders
2. Pirate ship
3. Tilt-A-Whirl
4. Pretzel

Immediately, Jonah's mood brightened. He kept asking to look at the list and to add to it. Now, every morning when we wait in the car at the bottom of our quarter-mile driveway for Erika and Hilary's bus and Jonah's van, Jonah amuses himself by typing his dream list on my iPhone:

1. School
2. Drive to waterpark and roller coaster park in Mr. Boss's car
3. Ketchup and French fries
4. Brown roller coaster
5. White roller coaster
6. Sesame Place
7. Beach
8. Swimming
9. Mall

Today's list had read:

1. Doctor
2. Pretzel
3. Chips
4. Spin around
5. Back room (code for any closet or other tight space
   where Jonah can chill and watch his iTouch)

I should note that the lists we make with Jonah aren't always followed to the letter; we wouldn't give him chips right after a big soft pretzel, but a boy can dream, right?

We're unable to find a pretzel—not in the cafeteria, the Starbucks station in the lobby, or even at the pastry cart parked in front of the hospital. The vendor informs us that the "pretzel guy" doesn't appear until about eleven o'clock. I grab a piece of coffee cake, another favorite of Jonah's, and hope that will suffice, along with two bottles of Crystal Light Lemonade, and we find our way back to the PACU.

Jonah is asleep when we get back. Liz informs us that they had to give him a dose of Versed because he woke up agitated and tried to pull off his oxygen mask. They just need to keep him still while they check his vital signs a few times. I sit by his bed, stroking his hair, intensely curious about the other patients in the eleven beds lining both sides of the PACU. Mostly, they are old, which doesn't surprise me. As I've mentioned, ECT is performed primarily on the elderly. There's one young Asian woman, who is accompanied by another young Asian woman. Other than that, the patients are alone. It all seems so routine, so singularly matter-of-fact, it's hard to reconcile this scene with the claim I've seen repeated in numerous places that ECT is the most controversial procedure in all of medicine.

In just a few minutes Jonah stirs. Liz instantly removes his IV before he pulls it out himself. As he opens his eyes, and struggles to sit up, Andy asks, "Jonah, what's Number 1?"

"He won't remember," I scold Andy under my breath, reminding him about the amnesia that Dr. Kellner warned us to expect. I assumed Jonah would remember nothing about these trips to Mount Sinai, maybe nothing from a month or two before or after. Not that there's any way to tell what Jonah remembers.

"Doctor," Jonah mutters groggily.

"Number 2?" Andy asks.

"Pretzel," Jonah manages to get out.

I'm stunned. My immediate reaction is to wonder whether the stimulus Dr. Kellner used was strong enough to provoke a therapeutic seizure. When he comes in to check on Jonah, he assures me that everything went perfectly. People vary greatly in their immediate response to ECT, we're told. Kids tend to recover from the anesthesia more quickly—like Jonah, who is already ready to leave while many of the adult patients who were treated before him are still in their beds. He's definitely unsteady, but Liz tells us we can go as long as we're careful. She knows it would be hard to keep Jonah in the bed if he didn't want to stay.

Andy and I get Jonah settled in the car with his blanket. Surprisingly, he doesn't want any lemonade. But he does want his pretzel.

"How about coffee cake?" I say.

"Pretzel," Jonah insists.

We have to drive Andy back to his office in midtown anyway, so we keep our eyes peeled for one of the seemingly thousands of pretzel vendors we encountered last night on our way back from the park with Jen. Naturally, now that we want one, there are no pretzels to be found. Andy double-parks while I run into a bakery that seems promising, but I discover it has no pretzels. Finally, we spot a pretzel stand on a corner. I hop out of the car while the traffic light is fortuitously red and wave dollar bills in my hand. The vendor smiles at me and places one of the gigantic twists in a little oven, but I point to our minivan, idling at the light, and yell that I have no time. It's too bad: the pretzel really is cold. But Jonah eats it anyway and seems happy.

On the way back to Andy's office where he will work the rest of the week, I ask him what he thought about ECT. He calls it a "non-event," referring not to the benefit we hope Jonah will gain from it, but to the quick and painless procedure, as well as Jonah's seemingly immediate recovery. I tell him about a study I read in which half of ECT patients surveyed considered going to the dentist worse than getting ECT.[1] This doesn't surprise him at all.

Getting out of town from Andy's office should be easy, even for someone as unfamiliar with Manhattan geography as I am: straight up 55th Street to 9th Avenue, which will take me right to the Lincoln Tunnel. But the Saint Patrick's Day Parade has streets blocked off and traffic snarled. Jonah and I both begin to get agitated at the jams and detours. "Aren't you supposed to be sleeping?" I ask, more to myself than to Jonah. I thought ECT was supposed to leave him groggy, possibly confused or disoriented. One mom told me her son slept most of the afternoon after his treatments. But Jonah, an hour or so post-ECT, seems totally fine.

"You should lie down," I tell him. "It's going to be a long trip home."

Jonah adjusts the blanket I brought along just for this purpose, but remains upright. "Coffee cake?" he asks.

I laugh. "No, you picked pretzel. We'll save the coffee cake for later." Jonah, being one of those immediate gratification types (kind of like me), isn't thrilled with this compromise. And he isn't happy about our creeping pace or the fact that I won't let him have my iPhone to type one of his lists. (If someone calls while he's using it, he just hangs up.) But all he does to show his irritation is squawk a few times: no banging on the windows, no kicking the seats, no lunging at me. I would have been more concerned had there been no agitation whatsoever in what is clearly an unpleasant situation. We're not looking, after all, to turn Jonah into the Stepford child.

MARCH 18, 2010

Liz Muller, the ECT nurse, calls to check and see how Jonah is doing. I tell her that he seems fine, very happy. I tell her that he's had no misbehaviors since before his ECT yesterday. I also tell her that I had expected Jonah to be groggy following his ECT and had been prepared for him to spend the rest of the afternoon sleeping. In fact, Jonah hadn't napped at all and seemed back to his normal (read high) energy level by the time we got back from Mount Sinai. "Is that what I should expect tomorrow?" I ask.

"Sometimes patients don't react much to the first ECT," Liz says. "Tomorrow's treatment will be much more indicative."

I hang up the phone, go downstairs, and announce to Keri, "ECT is just like pot!"

We laugh, because my one and only encounter with pot was the time I smoked it with Keri and one of our uncles, and it did absolutely nothing for me. This doesn't stop Andy from teasingly calling me "druggie" from time to time, since he has never experimented with pot or any other illicit substances. By comparison, my one afternoon at Uncle Ronnie's Florida ranch makes me a wild child.

"Did you tell the nurse that?" Keri wants to know.

"Of course not," I snort. I lean back against the counter, almost bent over in hysterics. It really isn't that funny, but it feels so good to laugh.

CHAPTER 6
Gary and David

I consider myself to have a finely tuned autism radar: if there's an autistic kid in the room, I can pick him out in half a second. But after meeting Gary and David (twenty-five), I found myself wondering if, in fact, I would have pegged them as being on the spectrum had I not already known. Although exceedingly soft-spoken and reluctant to converse, the twins have none of the distinguishing features I've seen in so many autistics: no bizarre hand movements, no obvious fixations. They just come across as extremely shy. It's easy to understand why their parents, Vicky and Bill, always assumed the twins would graduate from college and pursue careers. Perhaps Gary, the more compassionate one, would follow his interests in science and medicine to a job in physical therapy; maybe David would work with computers or accounting.

They are still hoping. Though the twins are doing great, from my perspective as a parent of a more severely afflicted child—Gary has his driver's permit, while David has already earned his license—they never did graduate from college. Their educational and professional plans were derailed almost ten years ago by debilitating episodes of catatonia and depression that Vicky believes threatened to land Gary—and perhaps David as well, although he was less profoundly impaired—in a psychiatric hospital, perhaps permanently.

———

Gary and David are fifteen years older than Jonah and his peers, so when I met the family I couldn't resist the impulse to ask Vicky about what life was like "back then." As a matter of fact, she smiled, she did have an ultrasound and found out she was pregnant with twins the same way I did: two fluttering heartbeats on a computer screen. She and Bill were overjoyed at the additions to their family, which already included two-year-old daughter Stephanie. And even though Gary and David were diagnosed in 1987, well before the dramatic increase in autism coverage and services that marked the start of the twenty-first century, Vicky's early observations of their development also sounded very familiar.

"When they were two, they weren't that interested in other kids," she told me, as we sat at her kitchen table eating bagels. "If I wanted them to play, I would have to sit on the floor with them and facilitate."

By the time Gary and David were three, their sometimes bizarre utterances had also begun to concern Vicky. "Not everything they said made sense," she said. "If you asked, 'Do you need to go to the bathroom?' they might say, 'I want to go to McDonald's and ride on the horse.'" They also exhibited some hand clapping and strange sounds, including grunting. Still, the idea the boys might be on the spectrum never occurred to Vicky or Bill: "How could they be autistic?" Vicky remembered thinking. "They hug, they're affectionate." It was the exact same logic Andy and I used to repeat to one another before Jonah's diagnosis, the mantra echoed by so many parents of autistic children I've met since then. For a public that has been, until very recently, educated in autism solely by the movie *Rain Man*, the tactile-defensiveness of Dustin Hoffman's character has come to define the disorder. Actually, although they virtually always have at least some difficulty socializing with peers, many autistic children are extremely loving and engaged with their parents and other important adults in their lives.

Vicky's path followed the same landmarks we would visit fifteen years later: an evaluation from a county therapist; confirmation from a developmental pediatrician; enrollment at an intervention preschool. And although the twins' diagnosis preceded by more than a decade the explosion in alternative therapies that recently culminated in Jenny McCarthy's controversial and very public proclamation that she had cured her son's autism with vitamins and a special diet, Vicky, as I did, researched extensively, pursuing every promising lead in her quest to heal her boys. Twice—once when Gary and David were in preschool and then again when they were in kindergarten—she flew to California to consult with Dr. Sydney Walker, the director of the Southern California Neuropsychiatric Institute and author of *A Dose of Sanity: Mind, Medicine and Misdiagnosis* and *Hyperactivity Hoax: How to Stop Drugging Your Child and Find Real Medical Help*. Dr. Walker appealed to Vicky because he believed he could find a physiological explanation for the boys' behavior.

"He decided that David was slightly hypoglycemic and thought that Gary might have epilepsy," Vicky told me. "But the epilepsy medication knocked him out. I brought him to a local doctor who gave him a twenty-four-hour EEG, and it turned out whatever Dr. Walker saw was just a movement artifact."

The failed regimens of Dr. Walker were followed by experiments with organic diets, gluten-free diets, B12 injections, and an odd cocktail of Bonine, Ritalin, and DHA. When they were in elementary school, the twins did three years of visual training with a therapist who had worked with professional hockey players. They also did brain training with a doctor who promised to make them normal by sitting them down for four hours every Sunday to trace squiggles on paper, play memory games, and write down one hundred uses for tissues. "He was so expensive," Vicky said. "And all that happened was that David broke Gary's tooth with a chair."

Listening to Vicky catalogue her ceaseless efforts over the last twenty years, I was awestruck yet again—as I have been with every parent I've talked to about ECT—at her dedication, her self-sacrifice, her sheer, unflagging, perseverance. This is why I find it so difficult to wrap my mind around anti-ECT comments, such as those that sprouted up all over the web following author Ann Bauer's revelation that her nineteen-year-old son's recovery from autistic catatonia—which she had previously reported without explanation, prompting a flurry of correspondence pleading with her to reveal exactly *how* this drastic improvement had transpired—was actually due to ECT. For example, one poster to the website NowPublic issued a clarion call demanding "the immediate public shaming of, and lawsuits for abuse, against Ann Bauer." These accusations of bad parenting truly defy logic when levied against parents whose commitments to their children—in terms of time, money, and emotional energy—border on the superhuman. And no, I'm not ringing my own bell here. I certainly don't include myself in this impressive group. Without the incredible level of support I've had since Jonah's diagnosis, I imagine I would have planted Jonah in front of the TV and drunk myself into oblivion years ago.

It wasn't just Vicky's pursuit of different therapies for Gary and David that impressed me so much. As doctor after doctor failed to deliver, she came to rely on the only thing that did seem to work:

constant and direct involvement with all aspects of her sons' lives, including school, activities and friends. Yes, friends: something many parents of autistic children, including myself, long for for our kids, while understanding it probably isn't anything they'll ever care about. Vicky volunteered with the Special Education PTA until the boys graduated from high school, serving the majority of those years as its president, primarily to meet the parents of the other students in the Special Education program. She set up playdate after playdate—most of which, she fully admitted, were utter failures.

"Playdates with typical kids don't work because the kids are so different," she said, preparing plates for Gary and David, who had just come downstairs after sleeping in all morning. "And Special Ed playdates don't work because the kids have different difficulties and different interests."

But a few of the playdates did work, and between those carefully facilitated exchanges and the countless teams and activities the boys participated in—including soccer, hockey, baseball, lacrosse, bowling, and boy scouts—the twins did make some friends. In fact, by fifth grade Gary and David were doing so well Vicky was able to resume working full time as a reading specialist, after working only part-time for the previous two years and not at all while the boys were younger.

"They had friends, they were busy all the time, just like regular fifth graders," Vicky told me. "David was in a blended class, so he was pulled out for English with a Special Ed teacher; Gary was in a regular class with a resource room. We always tried to separate them whenever possible because they're so codependent, but there weren't always appropriate classes." She smiled, describing how David would never initiate a conversation, but let Gary "boss him around."

The twins continued to thrive through ninth grade, the year, Vicky said, "they were at their very best, pretty close to typical for their age. They resembled learning disabled students more than kids on the autism spectrum."

Then at the end of their sophomore year of high school, everything started to fall apart. Gary began "freezing"—he would abruptly stop mid-stride, mid-meal, whatever he was doing, and he would remain stuck until someone tapped him on the shoulder. Always a good student, suddenly he was struggling. It took him six hours to complete a statewide standardized test for which his classmates were only allotted three hours. Although he passed the test, the aftermath was catastrophic.

"The test took so much out of him, he suffered a complete break," Vicky said. "After that day, he stopped talking altogether."

For over eighteen months, no one could figure out what was wrong with Gary. One doctor thought the bizarre symptoms were just part of his autism; another thought it was schizophrenia; yet another thought it was obsessive-compulsive disorder. He was prescribed antipsychotics, then antidepressants, but his behavior just kept getting worse. Periods of stupor were followed by periods of rage in which Gary would hit his sister, Stephanie; put his fist through the wall; even attack his mother. David, who rarely talked about his feelings, was distraught. "What's wrong with Gary?" he asked Vicky repeatedly, but she had no answers for him.

One thing she did know, as the twins' junior year in high school began, was that their public high school, with its thousands of students and inclusion program that had seemed so perfect for Gary, was no longer an appropriate placement for him. Vicky found an Alternative Learning Program (ALP) that agreed to accept Gary, but only for an hour or two a day.

"They wanted to help me because they could see I was desperate," Vicky explained. "But they just didn't think he could last the whole day." She cast a glance into the dining room, where Gary and David were finishing their breakfast, to see if they needed anything; Vicky had told them they could come in and meet me once they were done eating. "I was working full time. I had no choice but to let him come home and stay home alone." When Vicky returned, she would often find Gary frozen on the lawn by the basketball hoop. If Bill was still at work she would call her brother-in-law to get Gary in the house. She was too afraid he would get violent if she tried to move him.

It wasn't until Vicky and Bill took Gary to well-known psychiatrist and researcher Dr. Donald Klein that he was diagnosed with medical motor catatonia. Vicky was bewildered; she had always associated catatonia with schizophrenia. But new research suggests that up to 17 percent of autistic children will go on to develop catatonic symptoms in their teens.[1]

"Dr. Klein told us to go for ECT right away," Vicky said. "Just the sound of the words put me off. We hadn't done any research, we just knew all the traditional horror stories, where people shake."

Although Dr. Klein explained to them that ECT is done under general anesthesia, when he told them Gary might need as many as twenty treatments, they balked. Instead, Vicky and Bill opted to try Dr. Klein's second option: drastically increase Gary's dose of the anti-psychotic Geodon to "shock his system." But the larger dose made him sleep all the time.

Gary struggled along on a lower dose of Geodon for a while until his doctor prescribed lorazepam, which helped to some degree. "But he wasn't really back," Vicky explained. "He couldn't sit still; there was a lot of pacing. He couldn't focus on his schoolwork." But at least his behaviors had improved to the point where he was able to stay at his Alternative Learning Program all day, which seemed to Vicky and Bill like a step in the right direction. And then David, who had been thriving in school as an honor-roll student began to deteriorate as well. His symptoms first presented as depression: abandoned first by his twin, who had withdrawn into the world of catatonia, and then by his friends, as the gulf between their enormously complex social networks and his own limited ability to navigate them became increasingly obvious, it was hardly surprising to his parents that he was growing anxious and unhappy. Vicky first took David to a neighborhood psychologist but realized very quickly that the social and communication impairments endemic to autism make psychotherapy impossible. Next she tried antidepressants, which were similarly unsuccessful. So David also was moved out of his mainstream classes—although he was able to stay in the public high school, albeit in smaller, more supported "lab" classes.

That June, Gary and David graduated: Gary from his ALP, David from the public high school. But it was hardly a cause for celebration. "There were no jobs, no places for them," Vicky told me. "We just didn't know what else to do but send them to college." Although they found a transitional program at the New York Institute of Technology for kids with disabilities, Gary continued to struggle. "They called me every five minutes because of his bizarre behavior," Vicky said. "He wouldn't follow the schedule or follow directions; he was never in the place he was supposed to be at the right time. Basically, they threw him out by the end of the summer."

Vicky called Dr. Klein to report that the lorazepam wasn't helping enough. "He snapped, 'I told you to call Dr. Bailine,' and hung up," she said, referring to Dr. Samuel Bailine, the ECT doctor. Gary had been suffering from catatonia for three years at that point, and David had also begun exhibiting the "freezing" so characteristic of the disorder, although not to the same degree that his brother did. Vicky and Bill had done everything they could to avoid the ECT they had been bluntly informed was their son's best hope. There was nothing left to try.

———

Vicky keeps a scrapbook of highlights from the twins' lives. She, Gary, David, and I looked over it together. Vicky proudly pointed out the "Nicest to Know" award Gary was awarded in elementary school, the certificates the boys received when they earned their green belts in karate, their prom pictures. "Who is this?" she asked David, pointing to his date. "Didn't you go to two junior proms that year?"

There are no mementos from the ECT that both twins received when they were eighteen years old. I asked Gary what he remembered about those weeks. He said, "After the ECT, I felt better."

But Vicky's memories were somewhat less benign. "It wasn't easy to get him to go," she told me. "He would lock himself in the bathroom, and Dr. Bailine would have to chase him around."

I was interested to explore Gary's antipathy toward the treatments, since the issue of involuntary ECT pops up repeatedly in anti-ECT literature, even though the incidence is very small. California, one of the few states that closely monitors ECT use, reports that only 3 percent of the patients who receive ECT are forced to do so against their will. This statistic confirms Surgeon General David Satcher's assessment in his 1999 report on mental health: "In every state, the administration of ECT on an involuntary basis requires such a judicial proceeding at which patients may be represented by legal counsel. As a rule, such petitions are granted only where the prompt institution of ECT is regarded as potentially lifesaving, as in the case of a person who is grave danger because of lack of food or fluid intake caused by catatonia."[2] Or, as Vicky put it when I asked her if she ever considered cutting Gary's course of ECT short, "You can't live with someone who's violent and not verbal and doesn't eat. He'd be dead!

He couldn't go out with his brother to play basketball, or work, or do anything. When he was in that state, he couldn't make decisions."

I gently tried to ask Gary if there was a reason why he didn't like ECT. "Not really," he shrugged.

"Did it hurt?" I asked.

"It was a little painful, then I went to sleep. A little headache afterwards, that's it."

"Would you be upset if you had to go for ECT again?" I pressed.

"I wouldn't be upset," he said, in his soft voice.

David—who was also given ECT after Gary showed such tremendous improvement—reported a similar tale. He woke up from each treatment with a headache, but "It made me happier."

And it did make both boys happier, despite Gary's reluctance to go. ECT stopped the freezing, the rages, the depression. Both twins were able to return to school, where they earned certificates in Computer Business Operations. David continued on to a technical college where he completed a course that qualified him as a Physical Occupational Therapy Aide, including a certification in infant-adult CPR. In 2008, they were hired as recreation assistants at an assisted living facility where they were responsible for setting up games, serving snacks, and transitioning residents between activities. They became active once again in the community, including mentoring a severely autistic boy whom they took to the Y to play basketball. Vicky was no longer crying all the time. Her boys were back on track.

Naturally, this was when everything fell apart all over again.

This time, it wasn't anything ECT could help. In January 2009, Gary was diagnosed with Hodgkin's Lymphoma. The treatment, which included six months of chemo followed by forty radiation treatments, left him so withdrawn that Vicky wondered if she should call Dr. Bailine again—until he called her. Although the twins hadn't seen him for five years—completely contrary to the experiences of all the other families I've spoken with, maintenance ECT was never recommended for them, and their catatonia has remained at bay— he wanted to see how Gary and David were doing. When Vicky told him that Gary wasn't doing well, Dr. Bailine advised her to wait it out. Gary had, after all, been through a lot in the past few months.

My visit with the family occurred seven months after Gary's last radiation treatment, and Vicky felt he hadn't yet recovered completely. "He's still very quiet," she told me, after we had closed the scrapbook and the twins had left the kitchen to get ready to go to the gym.

Still, she and Bill were optimistic about their sons' future, even considering more independent living arrangements for Gary and David, although funding for housing for the disabled had been frozen in their state for the next three to five years. I told Vicky about JCHAI, a Philadelphia organization my husband works with that does exactly that: provides supported living arrangements for adults with disabilities, and she was very interested. It turned out her older daughter, Stephanie, was planning on moving to Pennsylvania shortly after her upcoming wedding. It put Vicky's mind at ease to imagine the twins living close to Stephanie, who had been so moved by her brothers' struggles growing up that she became a speech language pathologist.

In the meantime, Gary and David had some practice separating from their parents. In January 2010, they went to Israel on a birthright program. They had never been so far away from home for so long, and although Vicky was anxious the entire time they were gone, the twins had an amazing trip. Vicky showed me pictures: Gary on a camel, David with a new friend in a Jerusalem restaurant.

"Yes, they lead interesting lives," she agreed. "Now they're ready to lead independent lives."

CHAPTER 7

Jonah,

March–April 2010

ONE STEP FORWARD,
TWO STEPS BACK

MARCH 19, 2010

After another terrible night's sleep, my alarm goes off at four thirty a.m. This time I have new culprits on which to blame my insomnia: anxiety about sleeping through the alarm, driving up to Mount Sinai with Jonah by myself since Andy is still in New York, or how Jonah might survive a two-hour car ride with nothing to eat or drink. Now what I'm really afraid of is that I'm going to fall asleep at the wheel.

At ten minutes to five, I wake Jonah, guide him to the bathroom, and help him pull on pants and a T-shirt. I'm hoping he'll go back to sleep in the car, so I settle him in the last row of my mini-van with his favorite blanket and tell him to lie down. It's still dark outside, so I'm hoping he'll be fooled into thinking it's the middle of the night.

No such luck. Jonah immediately asks for his iTouch. I give it to him, steeling myself for what I expect will be two hours of endless and increasingly emphatic demands for lemonade, turkey, dates, pineapple, peanut butter sandwich: his typical breakfast fare. I was even careful not to pack snacks for later and nothing for myself but a much-needed cup of coffee (which I know he would never touch). I fully anticipate Jonah will tear the car apart looking for something, anything, to eat or drink. The lithium he takes, being a salt, makes him very thirsty, and although we held the lithium last night on Dr. Kellner's orders, Jonah just isn't used to waiting two hours for breakfast.

But the ride is surprisingly, shockingly, uneventful. I had also been concerned that Jonah would object once he found out we were going back to "the doctor's" as I had explained to him, assuming he wouldn't want another IV. But I promise him another pretzel once we're finished, and he doesn't say another word about food or complain about the doctor for the entire trip. I wonder if his agreeable disposition has anything to do with the ECT. All I can say for sure is that he hasn't had an aggressive outburst since before his treatment on Wednesday: not at school, not at home.

The sun is just beginning to rise when New York comes into view, the sky lightening into faint bands of blue and green. Again, I can't resist taking this beautiful skyline as a sign, re-imagining daybreak as a new beginning for Jonah. The traffic is light going through the tunnel, and we pick up Andy as scheduled before heading uptown to Mount Sinai. Although child patients typically have to be present at registration, Liz has cleared it with administration so that Andy can take Jonah straight up to the PACU while I complete the necessary paperwork. When I come without Andy, she tells me one of the orderlies can take Jonah up (if Jonah is comfortable with that) or I can walk him up, then come back down and register once he is sedated. I'm overwhelmed by the care and concern the ECT team continues to show for Jonah. All they want to do is make the process as easy as they can—both for him and for us.

By the time I find my way back to the PACU, Jonah is already unconscious. Everything goes pretty much as it had on Wednesday; Jonah wakes up within minutes of being wheeled back to his little recovery cubicle. Andy and I don't even make it down to the cafeteria, the whole process happens so quickly, and we're discharged by eight thirty. I had instructed Andy to bring a pretzel with him this time, but he was unable to get his hands on one, so we're in the same boat we were in on Wednesday. It seems ridiculous to me that the hardest thing about ECT thus far is finding a freakin' pretzel in New York at nine o'clock in the morning. We make it all the way back to Andy's office without seeing one vendor, but there's a gourmet food shop next door. Andy ducks in and comes out with . . . score! Not only does he have a pretzel, but he also brings a wedge of frittata for me. I hadn't even realized how starving I was until I opened the plastic container.

The drive home goes quickly. I hate driving in the dark, so just traveling through the sunny morning makes the return trip much easier. Jonah, like last time, is completely wide awake and seems perfectly happy.

Shortly after I cross the Pennsylvania border, Keri calls. "What are you doing when you get home?" she asks.

"Nothing," I say. "Just chilling with Jonah, I guess. Why?"

"They're closing the Toys"R"Us in King of Prussia," she tells me.

"What? Why?"

"They're knocking it down and building a gigantic new one," Keri says. "Anyway, they're clearing out the store and everything is on sale. I was wondering if you wanted to go."

I don't do a lot of shopping for myself—how many T-shirts and track pants, my typical wardrobe, can one person realistically be expected to go through each week? But I've always loved shopping for the kids. When Jonah and Erika were babies that obsession took the form of a severe Gymboree addiction. I literally couldn't walk through the mall without ending up with at least one tiny ensemble, complete with matching socks. Now that the kids are older, I seem to have been cured of that particular habit—Jonah, Erika, and Hilary all have adopted my exceedingly casual style. ("You must be so proud," Keri mused one morning as Erika trotted off to school in a pair of yoga pants and a hoodie.) And the twins have inherited so many clothes from their older siblings and cousins that I just can't justify the incredible shopping sprees I used to undertake every season.

But I'll never stop shopping for toys. There's always a reason. I have a cabinet I like to keep stocked with gifts for all the birthday parties the kids get invited to, but today I have a more pressing need: Erika's birthday is just two days away. Although I have the bulk of her presents, I wouldn't mind picking up one or two more, since instead of gifts she asked the girls attending her slumber party tomorrow night to bring pet food to donate to the local SPCA. I'm amazed by that kind of altruism in an almost-nine-year old. When I was that age, I never would have voluntarily given up the chance to get presents—heck, just two years ago, I wrote an essay for the parenting website Babble about how much I hate "no-gift" birthday parties, mostly because I believe kids deserve to be showered with useless crap one day a year. And damn it, Erika will be showered with useless crap, even I have to provide all of it myself.

Marina offers to give Jonah lunch while I go to Toys"R"Us with

Keri. The sale has only been going on for a couple of days, so the shelves are still relatively stocked. Everywhere I turn, I see something I want: a Lite-Brite for Hilary's birthday in May; a Polly Pocket set for Gretchen's birthday in June. For Erika, I'm excited to find an Arctic playset from Animal Planet that includes two mushers, a sled, and a pack of sled dog figures—her favorite kind of dog, which is her favorite kind of animal. But nothing gives me more pleasure than finding the perfect gift for Hilary: a Magic 8 Ball. Hilary is notorious in our household for constantly asking questions. Some I find incredibly profound, like, "What's it like to be a grown-up?" or "Are more expensive things better?" Others tend toward the blindingly obvious: "Why do they call it a bathtub?" Keri and I laugh, imagining all the times we'll be able to tell Hilary to consult her Magic 8 Ball when she interrupts whatever critical thing we're doing to ask what we would do if people didn't have any skin.

Talk about a cathartic shopping spree. It just feels so good to be in a happy place like Toys"R"Us, surrounded by regular parents with regular kids who would never in a million years consider shocking their children's brains. It's a very congenial community, even if I do get irritated at times by what I consider manufactured concerns, like whether water bottles have too much PBA or if Miley Cyrus is a bad role model because she danced on a pole. That's why I'm glad I had other kids, even though I knew with each of my pregnancies (except Erika's) that my babies had an increased chance of developing autism. The world of autism can be celebratory at times. It can be joyous and funny. But most of the time it's frustrating, worrisome, and even despairing. And all the time, no matter the emotional tenor of the moment, it's hard work. I just don't have the endurance to live there every second of the day. My other kids give me entrée into that other world, that blessed, comparatively easy world that no one appreciates as much as those of us who move back and forth. My cousin has a five-year-old son with autism, and she and her husband opted not to have a second child because they were too afraid of having another one with special needs. I know their financial resources are considerably less than ours, and they have far less help, so of course I understand. But I think that if I never had the opportunity to supervise playdates, chauffeur to gymnastics or soccer, answer crazy questions, help pick out a Halloween costume, or teach gardening, baking, chess, drawing, tennis, anything and everything—if I missed out on all those typical experiences, I think I would be much more bitter. Now I would just call myself slightly bitter—in a good way, like chocolate.

MARCH 20, 2010

Saturday mornings are hard. Jonah generally wakes up about six thirty, with the other kids rising over the next hour. I try to let Andy, exhausted from a week of ten-hour to twelve-plus-hour work-days, sleep in. Keri and Matty are around most weeks, of course, and they are a huge help. Matty generally makes a luxurious weekend breakfast, like pancakes or crepes, with sizzling platters of sausage and bacon. Still, it's a crazy time: not only do I have to supervise Jonah, but I have to make sure all the rest of the kids are ready to leave for their swimming lessons at nine.

Many of these mornings do, however, pass without incident. Jonah can be counted on to entertain himself with his iTouch or my computer—I have many of his favorite videos on my hard drive—and then there's always YouTube. Jonah loves looking up all his favorite Sesame Street songs and skits. I was shocked at how many homosexual and scatological parodies of Ernie and Bert there are on that site; fortunately, if Jonah doesn't recognize the music, he just moves on. And he can be left unsupervised while he's watching as long as someone is guarding the kitchen. Even if he's just eaten five minutes before, he's always trolling for food.

Generally, if Jonah knows there are grown-ups in the kitchen, he contents himself with his videos for a while. But this evening is Erika's birthday party, so Keri has baked a tray of brownies for the sundaes Erika has requested in lieu of a cake (topped by Andy's amazing homemade ice cream). The pan is cooling on the counter, and Jonah keeps coming through the kitchen, trying to snag some. Finally, he scores: while I'm reaching for milk at the back of the refrigerator, Jonah quickly sticks his fingers in the pan.

"That's it! Out of the kitchen," I yell at him. Jonah doesn't want to go and starts yelling and biting his hand.

That SIB warrants an immediate time out, but we don't do time outs in the kitchen because it's not a very safe environment: too many hard, possibly hot, possibly sharp surfaces; too many cabinets Jonah could smash with one hard kick. So I guide Jonah out of the kitchen to the butler's pantry, then I say, "Jonah, sit down. You're in time out."

That's when he comes after me.

Hearing the words, "You're in time out," has often precipitated a burst of aggression. I'm not sure if it's because Jonah finds time outs so disagreeable (he just has to sit quietly on the floor for one minute) or if it's because he has nothing left to lose once we've given him our maximum punishment—which, I imagine, was the logic behind the enhanced time outs one of the behavior specialists we worked with when Jonah was in kindergarten added to his protocol. One required him to calmly pick up hundreds of pieces of paper before the time out was concluded, which were thrown back on the floor the second he engaged in any self-injurious or aggressive acts. Needless to say, some of these time outs went on for hours.

But that was pre-ECT. At least, I'd been hoping it was. But as I block Jonah's flailing punches with my forearm, I realize that we're not done yet.

Matty, who was making breakfast, is there in an instant to deflect Jonah's blows and re-direct him to the floor. It takes a few attempts, but it works, and Jonah calms down. He comes after me again about half an hour later; this time, Andy is there to manage the aggression. He ends up taking Jonah out to do shopping for Erika's birthday party. This is how they spend a significant portion of every weekend: stocking our pantry and refrigerator from big-box stores, wholesale markets, and the occasional trip to a plain old grocery store for a few specialty items. Andy often has an aide to accompany him, but this week there's no help. I find it almost heroic that Andy can do a $500 Costco shopping trip with Jonah all by himself. It's something I would never even attempt to try, although my hope is that ECT will soon change that.

MARCH 22, 2010

When the alarm rings at four thirty a.m., it feels routine, even though it's only the second time. I jump out of bed, throw on fleece pants and a T-shirt, and splash water on my face. Andy needs to be in New York for work anyway today, so I will have company on the way up; while he showers, I load the car with Jonah's blanket, a thermos of lemonade (which I hide so he doesn't try to sneak any during the drive up to New York), and one more thing: his backpack. Today, I plan to drive Jonah straight to school after ECT. By the time we got home after the first two treatments, Jonah was completely alert and cheerful—although I couldn't say the same for myself. There's no reason for him to miss so much school if he can be there by eleven thirty, attentive and available for learning.

Just like Friday's commute, the trip to Mount Sinai is uneventful. It's nice not to have to drive both ways—Andy takes the wheel for this leg. Jonah doesn't ask for anything to eat or drink, but he keeps pestering Andy for his iPhone, wanting to type out a list. I think he's hoping to negotiate another trip to the beach, where he and Andy had gone the day before.

Like last time, Andy takes Jonah up while I complete the registration forms, which have to be signed again before each and every treatment. By the time I make it up to the PACU, Jonah is lying on the gurney in the treatment corner, a huge smile on his face while the staff assembles for the IV insertion. This time they barely need to restrain him. I'm not really surprised; Jonah, like many autistic kids, has a very high tolerance for pain. I didn't think he was fighting against the IV because it hurt so much as because he had no idea what was being done to him. Now that the ECT procedure is familiar, he is much more comfortable.

While we wait for the nurses and the anesthesiologist to get ready, Dr. Kellner asks me how Jonah's weekend went. I tell him about Jonah's three aggressive outbursts—the two on Saturday and one Sunday morning, also over food. He was desperate for a piece of the blueberry buckle that Keri had put in the oven to feed the girls at Erika's slumber party.

"That's a good sign," he tells me. "When you see the patient improve, but then the effect wears off between treatments, that generally means we can expect significant improvements long-term."

"How many treatments will it take before he stops regressing in between?" I ask.

Dr. Kellner shrugs; it depends. "About five or six," he says.

The PACU is relatively empty today, but Liz tells me that more patients are expected later. We are out by eight thirty and even though we have to drop Andy off at his office, we still make it to school before lunch. It feels so good to stretch my legs as I walk Jonah to his classroom. It was raining off and on the entire trip back from New York, and I'm exhausted from the early morning, the crazy bad-weather traffic getting out of the city, and the hypervigilance necessary to successfully navigate down the New Jersey Turnpike at seventy miles per hour in a storm. If I can say one thing about ECT thus far, it's that we've seen no personality-altering effects, no dulling of emotion. The first thing Jonah does when he sees his teacher, Nick Boss, is go up to him and say the same thing he asks every day: "Water park and roller coaster park in Mr. Boss's car. Please."

I consider taking a nap when I get home, but these hours of relative peace before all the kids come home are so precious, I hate to waste them. Instead, I hop in the shower, then find a leftover hamburger in the fridge that I eat cold, dipped in ketchup. Feeling somewhat refreshed, I head out to run a few errands. At three o'clock, right after he puts Jonah on the van to go home, Nick texts me: "He was very happy today, a lot of stims, but no time outs." I appreciate the immediate feedback; I know Nick and the other teachers take data each day on the students' behavior, but I had told them how especially important it was to me now, during ECT, to know about every disruptive episode. We want to be able to come to an objective conclusion about whether, and how much, ECT improves Jonah's aggression. By the time Jonah goes to bed at nine o'clock, the sum total of his aggressive behaviors for the day is still zero.

MARCH 24, 2010

This morning, Keri drives with Jonah and me up to Mount Sinai. It's so nice to have company, especially during that dark, brutally early trip up. Mostly, it'll be just me and a whole bunch of trucks. And I hate trucks.

Despite the fact that my obviously possessed GPS directs us over both the Verrazano and Brooklyn Bridges to get to the Mount Sinai campus in Manhattan (I followed the first suspicious turn because I vainly hoped the GPS was showing me a shortcut), we still get Jonah to school by eleven. He seems totally alert, but I'm a wreck. All afternoon, I feel as though I'm struggling under an enormous load of bricks, it's that difficult to move. I try to take a nap, but I can't fall asleep. I'm a very light sleeper; light, noise, and my own frenetic mind all conspire to keep me awake.

Later, after Jonah gets home from school, I check his backpack for his data sheet from the day. He's had so few behaviors since starting ECT I'm shocked to see he had a time out that lasted more than twenty-three minutes. I text Jonah's teacher to see if he has time to talk, and he calls me back shortly. It did take Jonah a long time to calm down, Nick confirms, but the aggression was very low. He came after Nick one time; then, in a separate episode, he grabbed another teacher's shirt. But, he wants me to know, "The most notable thing we've seen since Jonah started ECT is a real reduction in aggression."

I'm satisfied with this. As much as I would like all Jonah's behaviors to be instantly gone, we're not even halfway through the acute ECT course yet. I asked Dr. Kellner when we saw him that morning how many more treatments Jonah would have to get, and he thought Jonah would need about ten total, although he cautioned us this was only a guess. I should probably just let myself be happy about how much he's improved in only four treatments. Keri keeps commenting about how happy Jonah has seemed to her since starting ECT, and it's true, I've seen none of the crying jags we used to see periodically. Jonah also hasn't exhibited much in the way of random, unprovoked agitation. One of his time outs at school was precipitated by Nick's refusal of one of Jonah's constant requests to go to the "water park and roller coaster park in Mr. Boss's car." It may not be a great reason, but it's a reason.

Before dinner, while Jonah is working with one of his aides, I finally get around to opening a link Dr. Kolevzon had sent me the day we met in his office. I had asked him if there were other therapies we might consider, and he wrote that a colleague of his had a patient who improved dramatically on a new protocol. I clicked through to a blog called autismtso.com, which lauds "A potential . . . treatment for autism's most difficult symptoms." On the home page, a father, Stewart Johnson, describes how he spent thirteen of his son Lawrence's sixteen years researching autism, desperate for anything that might remedy Lawrence's aggression, SIB, perseveration, agitation, and OCD. After experimenting with TSO, Lawrence is now symptom-free on a dose of 2,500 ova every two weeks.

Ova?

Johnson goes on to explain a theory that I've heard before, that our hygienic society is responsible for the increase in asthma, autism, and other auto-immune disorders, and he claims that it's the reduction of "helminths" in the gut that might provoke this auto-immune response.

Helminths? Another word I don't recognize.

It takes me a few minutes of reading and clicking on the various sections of the website to figure out that helminths are a type of worm. Basically, the treatment involves mixing 2,500 worm eggs into a drink, giving it to your kid, and replenishing every two weeks because this particular type of parasite can't reproduce in the human body.

I have to laugh. This doesn't gross me out at all—I know our bodies are literally crawling with millions of parasites of all different ilk—and a natural treatment such as this must have many fewer side effects than the psychotropic meds Jonah's been prescribed to treat the same symptoms. I'm definitely intrigued, and although I would never start a new therapy right in the middle of Jonah's acute course of ECT, I email Dr. Kolevzon for more information. Still, I imagine telling my friends about the thousands of worms I'm feeding Jonah and realize I managed to stumble upon the one thing in the entire autism armamentarium that might disturb them more than shooting electricity into his brain.

MARCH 25, 2010

I sit in the rocking chair on the landing, listening to Jonah tantrum in his room. I can tell from the smacks that Jonah is banging and kicking against the mat on his floor, but I'm waiting here anyway in case he attacks his aide, Amanda. I make it a point not to run to Jonah whenever I hear him pitch a fit because I don't want him to learn that whenever he wants me, he just has to go after his aide. But I also don't want anyone to get hurt. Amanda, at just under a hundred pounds, is no match for a raging Jonah. I spend a lot of time in this rocking chair, watching, waiting to see if I'm needed.

Jonah has been having a very rough night. He hasn't hit anyone so far, but he's been in and out of time out for the past half hour or so, with a lot of screaming, crying and fierce SIB. He hasn't bloodied his own nose yet, which I suppose is a good sign, as is his lack of aggression against Amanda. But he is pounding himself hard and is having a lot of trouble calming down.

Dr. Kellner had said that the ECT would wear off quickly in the beginning, Keri reminds me when I go down to the kitchen to collect Jonah's meds for the night: maybe all this means is that he needs the ECT he's scheduled to get tomorrow. But Dr. Kellner also said that by treatment five or six he should be able to make it between treatments without regressing. And tomorrow will be our fifth session.

Once his tantrum is over, Amanda helps Jonah through his bedtime routine while I get ready for tomorrow, packing lunch bags for the other kids and stacking them in the refrigerator so Keri won't have to scramble in the morning without me. I've already filled the car with gas and stashed a soft pretzel in the glove compartment for Jonah's post-ECT meal, sheepishly wondering as I did it why it took me so long to figure out such an obvious solution to the pretzel problem. Tomorrow will be the first time I'm doing the entire trip by myself, so it's even more important than usual that I am completely prepared.

When I can't think of anything else I can do ahead of time, I go up and send Amanda home, taking her place in the rocking chair and guarding Jonah's room in case he decides that what he really wants to do isn't go to sleep, but to sneak down the back staircase to the kitchen and eat a dozen cookies. But I don't hear a sound from his room; I think he's probably already asleep. Still, I rock. The chair is embossed with the University of Pennsylvania seal; Andy and I both went to Penn, so when we found the chair with its five dollar price tag at an estate sale we felt fate had presented us with a gift we couldn't refuse, even though it didn't really go with any of our furniture. It's funny, my relationship with fate: I believe, and I don't believe. Although I like to pride myself on being too rational for any sort of abstract, intentional power, I also can't help seeing meaning everywhere I look—like when our friends offered us a kitten they found under their chicken coop, unaware our ten-year-old cat had just been hit by a car; or when Andy and I decided, on a past birthday of mine, to spontaneously dash down to the theater to see if they had any seats left for that night's performance of *Phantom of the Opera*—and they were sold out, except for two fourth row center seats someone must have turned in at the last minute. Surely it couldn't be just an accident that Dr. Wachtel had mentioned an ECT patient in the context of a conversation about different medication options, and that even though she couldn't provide it for Jonah, a close colleague was available only two hours from us. Surely, I tell myself as I rock, not feeling sure at all, we wouldn't have gone so far down this path if it weren't the right one?

Tonight is the first time I've really thought that ECT might not work. Of course I know that nothing is ever guaranteed, but I think deep down I really believed that the biggest obstacles we would face on our ECT journey were logistical ones: the Mount Sinai ethics committee, transporting Jonah back and forth, finding a local provider for maintenance ECT. It never occurred to me that we would succeed in everything except actually improving Jonah's behavior longer than a day or so with each treatment.

I tell myself again that it is way too early to be so defeatist. Although Dr. Kellner had predicted Jonah would only need ten treatments, acute courses of ECT for some patients have stretched as long as twenty or more. He is obviously responding—overall, his aggression has plummeted both at home and at school since the first treatment, and even as agitated as he was tonight, he didn't hit anyone. All good.

Still, I rock. Downstairs, Keri and Matty go through some last minute preparations for their trip to Ireland tomorrow, but otherwise, the house is quiet. I know I should go to bed, since the alarm will go off at four thirty a.m. again tomorrow, but I can't stop rocking; can't stop watching Jonah's door; can't shake the terrible uncertainty of not knowing whether we are going through all of this for nothing.

Finally, I will myself out of the chair and go check on Jonah. He is asleep, his iTouch resting on the sheet under his sweaty hand. I slide it out, pausing to adjust his blanket. Often, when I'm standing like this I can't help thinking about a short piece I read years ago by Jonathan Shestack, who founded Cure Autism Now in 1995 with his wife, Portia Iversen, after their son was diagnosed. It was just a few paragraphs in a CAN newsletter, but I've never forgotten it. Shestack describes going into Dov's room to watch him sleep after a long day of managing disruptive behaviors, admiring his sweet face, and feeling wracked with guilt over his relief at the prospect of a few hours of peace. Before that, most of what I had read about autism was uplifting and life-affirming, like Emily Perl Kingsley's "Welcome to Holland," which compares parenting a child with disabilities to embarking on a trip to Italy but ending up in Holland instead—a place that has its own beautiful landmarks to appreciate, even if they aren't the same sights you hoped to see in Italy. To hear as committed a parent as Shestack admit that caring for his son sometimes left him exhausted and overwhelmed was deeply reassuring.

Thirty seconds later I'm in bed, willing myself to fall asleep instantly, so I don't waste one minute of the few hours standing between me and the alarm. Of course, that's completely counter-productive. My mind continues to race: *What if it doesn't work? What if we can't stop the aggression? What if he hurts one of the other kids? What do we do next?*

Finally, I roll over on my back and stare up at the ceiling. *It's okay,* I tell myself. *There's always the worms.*

MARCH 26, 2010

Now that I know exactly what to pack and the fastest route to take, my first solo trip to and from Mount Sinai is a piece of cake. I call Liz as soon as I park, and John the orderly is waiting for Jonah and me in the registration area.

Jonah doesn't fight the IV now that he understands the routine, but he still doesn't like it. When one of the doctors says, "Jonah, time to lie down," Jonah says, "No lie down." This is how he often expresses his displeasure, by tacking "No" on to whatever it is you've asked him to do that he doesn't want to do (as in, "No time for bed," "No eat your carrots," "No kiss goodbye"), but I've noticed that people who don't know him very well sometimes have difficulty understanding him when he talks. One of the common troubles people seem to have is not hearing the "No." In this case, the doctor thinks Jonah has just repeated, "Lie down."

"Yeah, lie down," the doctor agrees.

Then Jonah lets loose with one of his most contemptuous expressions: "No yeeahhhh," the 'yeah' dragged out in vicious mimicry, as if Jonah has never heard such fatuous simplicity, such vapid, thoughtless, insincere encouragement in his entire life.

And the kicker is that none of the half-dozen or so people surrounding Jonah's gurney really followed that interchange, including one of the participants. I'm not sure if that compounds the irony, or the tragedy, or if it makes some kind of grand statement about the isolation of autism, or what. I can't even decide if I want to laugh or cry. Typical.

Just then John comes to walk me back through the maze of Mount Sinai to complete the paperwork. Liz tells me Jonah will be just fine and I know she's right; he has been through this enough times to know I'll be there when he wakes up.

When I get back to the PACU, Jonah is still sleeping, so I get a chance to tell Dr. Kellner about his behaviors over the past two days.

He admits, "This isn't the trend we want to see." He wants me to call him later, as he always does, to give him an update. Part of me wants to grill him, to try to pin him down about the significance of these behaviors, whether he thinks that after his initial improvements, Jonah may turn out to be a non-responder after all. But part of me doesn't even want to bring it up. I can guess what Dr. Kellner will say—that we'll just have to wait and see—and I don't need any more doubt to cloud my weekend, which Andy and I are spending alone in Atlantic City. Later tonight, Amanda will take Jonah for a respite weekend at Camp Joy, a camp for children and adults with developmental disabilities, and Oat and Marina will watch the rest of my kids. Keri, Matty, and their kids are on their way to Ireland, where Matty grew up. After all these four thirty mornings, it will be great to have two nights of sleeping until I wake up—even though I'll probably wake up at seven anyway because I'm such an early riser. We'll eat out, play poker, and just spend some time together.

So I don't press Dr. Kellner. He's already answered me anyway: a brief spike in behaviors is not a problem, as long as it doesn't represent a trend. And we don't have enough data points yet to know whether these outbursts represent a spike or a trend.

MARCH 29, 2010

Another rainy morning. As if the trucks and the darkness aren't enough, I don't think I've driven up to Mount Sinai by myself one time when it wasn't raining.

Still, I feel pretty good. Andy and I had a nice, relaxing weekend at our shore house. We slept late, watched two movies, played some poker, and went out to a fabulous steak dinner. And just being by the ocean relaxes me. Even better, Jonah had a great weekend at Camp Joy. Amanda reports that he came after her only one time, and it was pretty half-hearted at that. Jonah did have a big meltdown Sunday night at Walmart, hitting Andy ten or twelve times, but overall, two aggressions over an entire weekend is a vast improvement over previous weekends.

I relate all this to Dr. Kellner when he asks about how Jonah is doing, and he asks me, "If we stopped right here, would you say that ECT was a success?"

I watch Jonah, calmly waiting on his gurney to be rolled to the ECT corner. "I would say it's been a definite improvement," I say. "But I'm not sure it's enough to change the course of things. Even one aggression per week is too much for him to live at home, especially as he gets bigger."

Dr. Kellner considers this. "I think we can get him better," he says. "I'm going to increase the charge today, since he's been handling the treatments so well. We'll go through the week and see how he does."

I get a little nervous as I go back downstairs to take care of the registration paperwork. Jonah has seemed completely lucid within an hour post-ECT; will it be different this time? What if Dr. Kellner goes too high?

When I return to the PACU, Jonah is still sleeping. I immediately start peppering Liz with questions until she tells me I should talk to one of the doctors. She gets Dr. Dennis Popeo, a younger colleague of Dr. Kellner's.

I ask Dr. Popeo about the increase in charge. "What are you giving him now, and what was he getting?" I ask.

Dr. Popeo explains that the maximum charge the ECT machine can administer is five hundred millicoulombs (mC), which is less than a third of that given to jolt the heart back into rhythm. He holds his hands up as if they're paddles and says, "Clear!" to make sure I know what he's talking about. He can't assume I've seen anyone treated for cardiac arrest, but it's a reasonable bet I've seen *Grey's Anatomy*.

"We talk about charge in terms of percentage of max," Dr. Popeo tells me. "We start everyone on 5 percent which is the lowest. That's where we started Jonah. Then we moved up to 15 percent when we saw how well he did. Today we went up to 20 percent. At some point we'll see a plateau in terms of benefit."

Jonah wakes up shortly after Dr. Popeo leaves. Liz is with him right away, removing his oxygen tube and IV before he can pull them himself, checking his vitals, having me sign the necessary papers so we can leave as soon as Jonah can pull himself off the bed—which usually happens within minutes of his awakening. No one else is in and out faster than Jonah. In fact, although some of the beds are occupied before we get there, no one leaves before we do.

When Jonah seems at least partially coherent, Liz usually asks me to go over the list we made on the way over. Number 1 is always "doctor;" Number 2 is always "pretzel." So those are easy to remember. Today, Number 3 is "blue juice"—a departure, since usually he has lemonade to drink, but yesterday Andy bought him a bottle of Gatorade as a post-ECT treat.

"What's Number 1, Jonah?" I ask.

"Doctor," he mumbles.

"That's right, Jonah! Now, that's done. What's Number 2?"

"Pretzel," he knows.

"That's right!" I say again. "And I have one waiting for you in the car. Now, Jonah, what's Number 3?"

Nothing.

"Jonah, what's Number 3?"

"Spin," he says, slowly.

Wrong answer. But he is still very groggy. Has the higher dose affected his memory? Or is he just still feeling the effects of the anesthesia, the seizure, the Versed? I shake my head with frustration at the near impossibility of determining whether Jonah is experiencing any significant side effects from ECT. Testing his memory is extraordinarily difficult, since he has a lot of trouble under the best of circumstances answering questions about anything but the present; he will tell me what he wants for snack, for example, but will ignore me if I ask, "What did you do at school today?" Memory lapses would be more apparent at school, where much of Jonah's table work focuses on building his vocabulary by learning the features, functions, and classes of different objects—requiring him to name the parts of a bug, for instance, or list six types of vehicles—but Nick hasn't reported any drop in his performance. As far as physical discomfort, Jonah never complains of nausea or headaches, but as I mentioned earlier, he has a very high tolerance for pain. The only time he has ever come to me for help is when he spilled a box of thumb tacks on the floor and hobbled to me with three or four stuck in the bottom of his foot, directing, "Fix it." So I suppose it's possible that he's experiencing headaches that I might find unbearable, but in the vein of the tree falling in the forest, if it doesn't bother him, can it be properly called a headache?

Liz, who's been wrapping things up, doesn't seem that concerned. "I'll call you later," she says, as Jonah stumbles out of the PACU.

MARCH 31, 2010

Today, I have some company on the way up to Mount Sinai: Andy has to be in the New York office, so he's coming with me to Jonah's ECT. I'll drop him off at the office afterward, then drive home. I need to come back tomorrow since Jonah's participating in a genetic study of Dr. Kolevzon's; the three of us will stay over at Andy's friend Adam's place, then continue down to our house in Atlantic City after Jonah's Friday ECT, which looks like it will be the last in his acute series.

Family members aren't allowed in the PACU during the actual treatment, so Andy and I cram ourselves onto a gurney in the hall and play Scramble on Andy's iPhone while we wait. After a few minutes Dr. Kellner comes out to let us know that Jonah had another successful seizure. I quickly exit the game and await his report.

First, he wants to know how much Andy and I feel the ECT has helped reduce Jonah's behaviors. Andy and I look at each other and shrug. Despite my initial concerns about the increased charge, Jonah still has shown no discernible memory loss, cognitive impairment, or personality change. Still, I find these types of subjective evaluations very stressful. I'm always afraid of not getting it exactly right and of treatment decisions being made based on my vague determinations.

"Aggression reduced by 85 percent?" I say. "More, probably."

"Definitely more," Andy agrees.

"SIB less," I say.

"Really?" Andy says.

"I think so." It seems as if Jonah has been engaging in a lot more "happy SIB"—biting his hand in excitement, not agitation.

"I ask because we're at a tough place right now," Dr. Kellner says.

"We want to go as far as we can go, but not too far—we want to use as much electricity as we need, but we don't want to use more electricity unnecessarily."

"Although that makes it more likely he'll get superpowers," Andy says, completely deadpan.

Dr. Kellner laughs, the first time I've ever heard him. He is usually warm, interested—but completely serious. Now he demurs, "We don't like to brag about that."

You gotta love ECT humor. Calling everything "shocking" is just the beginning.

Ultimately, we confirm that Friday will be Jonah's last treatment with Dr. Kellner, who has sent Jonah's records to a colleague, Dr. Richard Jaffe, at the Belmont Center for Comprehensive Treatment in Philadelphia—a mere twenty minutes from our house. Dr. Jaffe has agreed to provide the maintenance ECT that Jonah will need indefinitely. Dr. Kellner promises to email me Dr. Jaffe's contact information so I can set up our first appointment.

APRIL 1, 2010

Driving up to New York in the bright sunshine is much better than the early morning darkness, but I pay the price in traffic going through the Lincoln Tunnel. Jonah is patient as we stutter our way through.

"No doctor," he says.

"This is a different doctor," I tell him, trying to think of a way to explain it to him. "I know we're going to the same place where you get stuck with the needle, but this is a talking doctor. Nothing he does is going to hurt."

I'm very interested to see how Jonah does in today's testing session. We've agreed to participate in Dr. Kolevzon's genetic study, the first part of which is the Autism Diagnostic Observation Schedule (ADOS), a diagnostic tool. Since Jonah's been on spring break all week, this is the first time in seven days he'll be in anything even vaguely resembling a classroom where someone will be placing demands on him. The first time we met with Dr. Kolevzon, right before ECT, he tried just asking Jonah a few questions, and Jonah ended up having a tantrum on the floor of his office. I'm hoping today will look a lot different.

First, Dr. Kolevzon takes Jonah and me into an empty office to reassess Jonah's compulsive behaviors, using the Children's Yale-Brown Obsessive Compulsive Scale (CYBOCS). Dr. Kolevzon had asked me to rate the magnitude of Jonah's SIB, spinning, list-making, and other compulsive behaviors pre-ECT, and now asks me the same questions again.

"Actually, I don't even consider list-making to be maladaptive," I said. "If it helps Jonah structure his day, then that's fine. I'm not going to try to get him to stop it."

Dr. Kolevzon crosses "list-making" off his sheet.

"His SIB is definitely reduced . . . he still hits himself quite a bit, but it's happy SIB, not agitated."

Dr. Kolevzon marks Jonah's SIB as "severe," rather than "extreme," my last rating.

"He still spins a lot, but again, he does that when he's happy."

When we're done, Jonah's score this time around is 44 percent lower than it was the first time. He also scores 25 percent lower on the Aberrant Behavior Checklist (ABC). "That's a significant improvement," Dr. Kolevzon says, impressed.

"Sure, but this is just based on my subjective evaluations," I say. "I really wish I had objective data."

When Jonah was on the NBU, every single aggression, every SIB, every disruptive behavior was noted on a clicker. This perfect data collection made it very easy to assess the efficacy, or lack thereof, of every medication change or new element of the behavior plan. Milagre, Jonah's school, is also good about taking data, but Jonah's been on break for seven days, right when we would really expect to see the most benefit from the ECT. I can say that his aggression is way down and that he seems to me to be much happier. Andy, Keri, Matty, Marina, and Jonah's aides can all agree with me, but when it comes right down to it, that's just a whole lot of overall impressions.

What I want to know, but don't ask, is what Dr. Kolevzon thinks of Jonah today. Instead of pitching a fit, Jonah's spent our entire time in Dr. Kolevzon's office trying to search YouTube on Dr. Kolevzon's impossibly slow computer. He's happy the whole time—no agitation, no aggression, a few happy SIBs, that's it. But my interview with Dr. Kolevzon is short, and before I know it Jonah and I are escorted to a testing room where another psychologist will administer the ADOS, which will be videotaped and then processed by multiple scorers to ensure reliability.

Jonah bounds happily enough into the testing room. His attention is momentarily drawn by a noisy Sesame Street toy on a small table, but none of the other toys scattered around hold his interest. He keeps asking for his iTouch back.

There are different sections of this test, which I remember vaguely from the last time Jonah had it done, when he was two and a half years old. Actually, the only part I really remember is the pretend birthday party: the tester sets up a baby doll and some toy plates, and asks about the steps of a birthday party. I think even back then Jonah got the concept of feeding the baby with the toy fork. He still gets it, but he's much more interested in eating the Play-Doh the psychologist has brought out to represent the cake—a modification since the test was last administered nine years ago. Jonah knows the Play-Doh isn't really cake, but he happens to really like Play-Doh. We stopped letting him play with it at home for just this reason. After he shoves a particularly large chunk in his mouth, the psychologist apologizes. "I'm sorry, I thought I could stop him in time."

That's what everyone thinks. No one really believes how fast Jonah is or how strong he is until they see for themselves. "It's okay," I say. "It's not toxic."

The part of the assessment that's most striking to me is one that none of the scorers will probably notice at all—that Jonah has no behaviors the entire time. He doesn't listen to the psychologist some of the time, and once he discovers the chips she has stored in the closet he perseverates on them to such an extent she agrees to move the "snack" portion of the test to, say, right now; still no agitation, no aggression. It seems fairly safe now to call the few aggressive behaviors Jonah's had since starting ECT blips, not a trend. The trend clearly illustrates substantial improvement—not just in the decrease in hitting, but in the overall lifting of Jonah's mood.

We're done with the test by three thirty. Our plan is to meet Andy, Jen, and her boyfriend, Matt, for dinner, but we have a couple of hours to kill until then. Feeling optimistic, I decide that Jonah and I should take a walk in Central Park, maybe go to the zoo. It's a beautiful day, sunny and seventy degrees outside, one of the first really perfect spring days of the season. Of course, I'm not the only person in

New York City to notice the weather. The park is mobbed—we can't even get close to the zoo, and just navigating the paths is difficult. I feel very anxious—I'm afraid of losing Jonah, and I'm afraid he's going to do something crazy, like jump in the pond (as we walk by, he turns to me and says, "Bathing suit"). It isn't long before I guide Jonah out of the park and to Andy's office, even though Andy still has two meetings before he can leave. I let Jonah watch YouTube in an empty office and collapse on a couch. But even as I lament our failed outing, I remind myself that this was altogether a different kind of failure: this was my failure, not Jonah's. It was my anxiety about the crowds, about everything that might go wrong, that drove us inside—not any misbehavior on Jonah's part. In fact, he seemed to mind the throngs of people less than I did. Once he got the soft pretzel I had promised him after the testing session, he was fine. I wonder how long it will take before I trust him.

Jen, Matt, Andy and I return to the same Outback we went to the last time we saw Jen. I'm very curious whether Jen will notice a change in Jonah, since she has weathered a lot of his tantrums over the three years she worked with him. And she does remark how much calmer he seems. But of course, she knows about the ECT. I remember Jonah's speech therapist never wanted to know whether we had changed Jonah's medications because she was afraid it would bias her perceptions of his behavior. I thought that was so smart, but it's one thing not to disclose a change in meds; it's another thing to introduce such a major, time-consuming intervention as ECT without alerting Jonah's teachers and therapists. What we lose in objectivity, I think as I cut into my rare filet, we make up in unanimity. Jonah's teachers, therapists, aides, former aides, doctors, family—we can't all be wrong, can we?

CHAPTER 8

Sam

On an ordinary day in June 2011, I met fifteen-year-old Sam and his mother, Susan, for coffee. Sam is an ordinary boy; a little brighter and a lot less contemptuous of adults than I, with my limited teenage experience, was expecting, but he liked ordinary things, like riding his bike, cooking, and watching movies. He worshipped his two older brothers and wanted to be a doctor when he grew up. In fact, unlike my outings with Jonah, where I feel we're under constant public scrutiny because of his clapping, bouncing, shrieking, spinning (and my constant refrain: "Jonah, don't touch that! Jonah, get back here!"), I bet not one of the dozens of people who walked past our table at that sidewalk café noticed us, we were all so ordinary. They would have done a quick double take, however, if they had overheard our conversation. Especially the part where Sam spoke of the paranoid delusions that used to keep him from leaving his house. "I thought people were listening and watching me," he said softly, embarrassed despite Susan's gentle reminders that his symptoms were in no way his fault. "I would spend hours adjusting the blinds. There was one perfect position where no one could see in, but some light could still come through." This was the most benign of Sam's episodes; the others—in which he tried to jump out a second story window, or believed the character from the Burger King commercials was going to come to his house and rape him, or stayed awake for four days straight—his mother had to tell me about. Like many patients, Sam didn't remember much from his psychotic periods. Although he did remember enough to add, "It doesn't feel like paranoia when it's you. It feels like real fear."

I sipped my coffee, trying not to intimidate Sam with my barely containable excitement. I'd met several boys over the past year whose lives had been transformed by ECT; unlike the others, though, Sam is completely neurotypical. He doesn't suffer from autism or any other developmental delay that would keep him from talking about his experience. Susan is an unabashed supporter of ECT, crediting it with saving her son's life. But I was dying to know: *What was it like for Sam?*

———

Sam's symptoms first appeared when he was in sixth grade. Initially, Susan and her husband, Rick, assumed it was the difficult transition to middle school that had left their son so depressed. School had never been easy for Sam, whose social and academic struggles had earned him an ADD diagnosis as early as first grade. Combined with his slight stature and shy demeanor, Susan and Rick wondered if Sam had become a target for his middle school peers, who, Susan acknowledged, "weren't always very nice."

But when Sam's general sadness deteriorated into fierce crying jags and suicidality, when he all but stopped eating and sleeping, Susan and Rick knew Sam was suffering more than growing pains. "We're not ashamed to seek help," Susan told me. "Those are our jobs." Susan is an ER nurse and Rick, a psychotherapist. After their son lost a quarter of his body weight, it was obvious to both of them that he needed more than their unconditional love and support.

Sam's three-year experiment with psychotropic medication began with a partial hospitalization. The goal of such a program—in which patients spend their days at the hospital, then go home to sleep—is to make rapid medication changes while under daily doctor supervision. But Sam never felt comfortable in the program. "The other kids weren't like me," he explained. "They were violent. Most of them were there for drug use or skipping school." And although Sam's symptoms improved slightly, Susan waited in vain for him to "get to a place where he was functional and well."

Sam's continued instability was exacerbated by brutal side effects from his medication. The worst was akathesia, typically described as feeling as though you have "ants in your pants." But when I echoed this phrase back to Sam, he interrupted me. "It's much, much worse," he said. "It's torture." The akathesia made him agitated and caused pacing, rocking, and scratching Sam had no control over. He continually poked himself with a pencil. His doctors responded to these behaviors by increasing the dose, which naturally made everything worse.

Sam suffered his first manic episode in July 2009 as a reaction to a new antidepressant. Selective serotonin reuptake inhibitors (SSRIs) frequently trigger mania in patients whose bipolar disorder has been misdiagnosed as depression; Jonah's bipolar was discovered the same way. It was a terrifying ordeal for the entire family. That was the time Sam—and Susan—didn't sleep for four days. Sam was plagued with gory hallucinations of bloody faces and heard voices of people all around him murmuring words he couldn't quite understand. Susan sat with him in his room, trying to calm him down, desperately trying to keep her eyes open. Sam couldn't be left alone even for a moment. The times she'd let her guard down, she found him with a jump rope around his neck or a knife to his throat. And Rick wasn't much help. Although he tried to spell Susan, offering to watch Sam while she went to the supermarket, he called her back immediately. He just had no idea what to do when his son began raving about the Burger King mascot or the poisons he was certain had been hidden in his food.

Susan and Rick had hoped to keep Sam home while they adjusted his medication, but ultimately they both agreed it wasn't safe. He was hospitalized for eight days while his psychiatrist struggled to stabilize his mood. Although the doctor did successfully treat Sam's psychosis, his behavior continued to be erratic even after his discharge. Susan began working only weekends so someone would always be home with Sam, who could vacillate between hysterical laughter and inconsolable sadness in the span of a few minutes. And he continued to suffer bad side effects from his cocktail. "One pill made me hungry all the time," Sam said. "I needed to eat until I almost threw up." He gained almost a pound a day until that prescription was discontinued. Other drugs gave him psoriasis, hypothyroidism, and metabolic syndrome, which can cause dangerously increased levels of cholesterol and blood sugar. He also experienced cognitive impairments so severe he was unable to complete even open-book exams. When he was in ninth grade, he completely forgot his multiplication tables.

The scariest complication came in March 2010, when Sam developed high heart rate, elevated blood pressure, agitation, and confusion. He was diagnosed with serotonin syndrome and hospitalized for three days while doctors weaned him off the offending drugs. Frustrated with their private psychiatrist, Susan and Rick were thrilled to discover that the psychiatrist on call the weekend Sam was admitted to the hospital was a national expert in child pharmacology. After Sam came home, they decided to switch to the new doctor for good. If anyone could handpick the exact formula out of the infinite combinations of drugs and dosages, surely it was a national expert in child pharmacology.

But even the expert was out of ideas. Sam had already been prescribed every medication typically used to treat bipolar disorder, including lithium, Depakote, and various antipsychotics, antiseizure medications, and antidepressants. Although he didn't know much about it, the expert suspected ECT was Sam's last and best chance to get well.

This was hardly what Susan and Rick expected to hear from the expert on pharmacology, and Rick was alarmed. All he knew about ECT were the dark rumors he had heard. He warned Sam about brain damage and memory loss. But Sam was intrigued. "So many meds gave me so many horrible side effects—one even made it hard for me to breathe," he told me. "I was just excited to try something different." He Googled ECT and read everything he could find, while Susan talked to anyone she could think of who might have any experience with ECT. All she heard from counselors, therapists—even the receptionist at one practice—were stories of dramatic improvements.

"We wouldn't have done ECT if Sam hadn't wanted to," Susan said. "He's a bright kid; I wouldn't have forced him." In the end, even Rick agreed that Sam, who was barely functioning, had nothing left to lose.

Sam's first ECT was scheduled in October 2010. Afterwards, he wound up in the hospital for three days with fever, confusion, and chest pain. Emergency room doctors suspected he had developed neuroleptic malignant syndrome from combining the general anesthesia he was administered during ECT with all the medications he was already taking. The local psychiatrist Susan had found to provide Sam's acute course of ECT, already uncomfortable treating such a young patient, refused to continue.

"That didn't make you want to stop?" I asked Susan.

She shook her head. "Because for those three days, after one treatment, Sam was the calmest, most well he had been in years. He wasn't happy to be in the hospital, but he wasn't anxious, not paranoid, not agitated. It actually made me more determined it would work."

But for a while it looked as though Susan's determination wouldn't be enough to get Sam the ECT she felt he desperately needed. Although the family lived outside a major city, not one of the local hospitals would agree to treat Sam because of his age. Susan persisted, expanding her search area ever wider until she found Dr. Kellner, about eighty miles away.

When Susan and I first exchanged emails, I had no idea her son was also a patient of Dr. Kellner's. Susan got in touch with me after reading a short post I wrote about our experience with ECT that was published online. We discovered the connection during our first meeting, which took place over lunch while Sam was at school. It was exactly like finding out that your hygienist or yoga instructor or veterinarian went to your high school. We commiserated over all those pre-dawn trips to Mount Sinai; we swapped stories about Dr. Kellner's dry humor and his love of fine restaurants; and we reminisced fondly about his nurse Liz, who, upon hearing that Sam wanted to be a neurologist when he grew up, presented him each week with an old neurology textbook she had dug out of Dr. Kellner's office.

Four months elapsed between Sam's first ECT treatment and his second, which was his first at Mount Sinai. Dr. Kellner asked Susan to wean Sam off all his medications to prevent another reaction like the one that landed him in the hospital. As a result, he was so psychotic and manic he could barely participate in the baseline mental exam Liz gave him to later assess whether his treatments had caused any cognitive impairment. Sam couldn't tell her what city he was in, who was the president, or what the date was. He couldn't draw a hexagon. Liz administered the test before each treatment, until Sam had recovered so significantly that he effortlessly nailed the questions every time.

But it took a while. "Sam's mania actually got worse after ECT for three or four sessions," Susan told me. "Dr. Kellner told me that might happen." Just like antidepressants, ECT can, in rare instances, provoke a manic state in patients with bipolar disorder. "But I was crying all the time. Sam wasn't improving, and I wasn't sleeping, and we were getting up at four a.m. to drive to New York, where Sam would try to get out of the car while we were moving because he thought the taxis were police cars coming to get him."

After the first week, Dr. Kellner switched from unilateral to bilateral ECT, a distinction that refers to the location on the head where the electrodes are placed. In bilateral ECT (BL), electrodes are affixed to both the right and left sides of the head, whereas in unilateral (RUL), the two electrodes are attached to the front and back of the same side of the head—typically on the right side. This theoretically spares the speech and language center, which is almost always found on the left side of the brain. Studies comparing the two placements have been published since the 1950s when RUL was developed in an attempt to reduce the short-term memory loss and disorientation some patients experienced after BL ECT.

Although studies did initially confirm that patients given RUL ECT reported slightly fewer side effects, they also found that RUL was significantly less effective than BL unless the electrical dosage was substantially increased to the now-standard six times seizure threshold—the amount of electricity required to elicit a seizure, typically about 75–150 mC, or roughly the current needed to light a 100 watt lightbulb for one second. This dose resulted in the same degree of cognitive side effects as BL ECT. In 2010, the Consortium for Research in ECT (CORE), led by Dr. Kellner, released the results of a randomized trial of the different electrode placements involving 230 patients from five treatment centers. The researchers concluded there were no differences among BL, high dosage RUL, or bifrontal (BF—a third electrode placement in which both electrodes are placed on the forehead) in either efficacy or degree of cognitive impairment. The only distinction they reported was that the BL ECT group showed the fastest improvement, which is why it has always been the preferred placement for acute patients who are actively suicidal or who suffer from potentially fatal conditions, such as catatonia.[1]

Or for those who fail to respond to RUL ECT. Doctors aren't sure why, but about 20 percent of patients fail to improve after even high-dose RUL. Sam was part of that group. His paranoia, psychosis, and mania began to resolve almost immediately following the switch to bilateral ECT. By March, he was well enough for what I've come to see as the gold standard for recovery in the families I've interviewed: the family vacation. The previous year, Susan and Rick had had to cancel a trip to Niagara Falls because Sam was so sick. In March 2011, the family spent a glorious week in Discovery Cove where Sam swam with dolphins who, he informed me, are so smart they can be taught to play poker.

————

      I'm not sure what I had expected from Sam, but I couldn't help feeling the slightest bit disappointed as I walked back to my car. Where were the flashing lights, the rushing hormones, that eye-of-the-hurricane perspective on ECT I had hoped to hear for the first time?

As I buckled my seatbelt, I shook my head at my own ridiculousness. Of course Sam couldn't describe the actual ECT procedure: he was, like everyone else, under general anesthesia. And his memory of those three weeks he drove back and forth to Mount Sinai for the acute course was cloudy. Susan mused drily, "He does forget the lobster tail lunch we had—we should have had McDonald's." What Sam did say with certainty was that he feared the IV more than any other part of the procedure, and that "getting a blood test is definitely worse."

Sam wasn't, however, at all fuzzy about how ECT gave him his life back. His academic performance improved, and he was happily enrolled at a small private school for kids who struggled in the enormous public high schools that, in Sam's district, each service about three thousand students. In school, Sam received both group and individual therapy while completing college prep-level classes and participating in community service, such as preparing meals for the homeless—a perfect project for him, since he loves to cook. He was also acting on his dream of a career in medicine by volunteering at a local hospital. "I'm just going to push the cart around and hand out things to patients or work in the gift shop," he said, a bit dismissively, but I could tell from Susan's smile what it meant for her family, that the boy who for so many years had needed so much help was now able to help others.

"It's been a real adjustment for me, going to having a well kid from having a sick kid," she said. "I'm still hyper-vigilant, afraid it's going to come back."

But there was no doubt in Sam's or Susan's minds about what they would do, should that happen. "Definitely," Sam said, when I asked him if he would get ECT again. "It's the best treatment I've had, with the least side effects."

———

In 2011, Sam was speaking hypothetically. He was healthy, stable, ashamed of the bizarre behavior that seemed, from his post-ECT perspective, as though it had been committed by someone else. But bipolar disorder isn't curable, and Susan was right to be vigilant. In May 2012, Sam's symptoms came back. The question of how to respond was no longer hypothetical.

This time around, Sam never progressed to the point of psychosis and hallucinations. Their experience managing their son's disease enabled Susan and Rick to recognize early, subtle indications. "We say we know the bipolar is back when Sam puts on his lab coat," Susan told me, referring to a cherished hand-me-down from her oldest son, now in medical school. "Sam wears an ID badge and walks around handing out business cards, saying he's going to be a world-famous neurologist. When he's too happy, too talkative—now we know those are early signs of mania."

Sam's doctor described his condition as a "mixed bipolar state," meaning Sam cycled rapidly through manic and depressive episodes. As charming as he was waxing about his Ivy League plans in his oversized lab coat, it wasn't long before he became angry and irritable, despondent about the prospects of ever getting into college. He would retreat into the house, close the blinds, and refuse to leave, sure that people were talking about him behind his back. Some days he was completely unreachable: pacing, ranting, laughing hysterically about nothing. He could no longer volunteer at the hospital where he had been helping nurses and patients for the past eighteen months. At his lowest, he wished aloud that he were dead.

Although a cocktail of the anticonvulsant Lamictal and the antipsychotic Geodon had kept Sam stable for the past year, it obviously was no longer working. "We gave Sam the choice," Susan said. "ECT, try new meds, or do nothing. It was important to us that at his age he had control over his medical decisions." To Sam, the choice was obvious: the medications made him fuzzier than ECT ever did. In July, he began his second acute course, followed this time by maintenance treatments every two weeks.

Just like the first time, Sam landed in the hospital with neuroleptic malignant syndrome after starting the acute course. His doctors agreed that his medications hadn't been discontinued early enough before the administration of general anesthesia, causing a dangerous reaction. Sam resumed ECT uneventfully once the medications were out of his system, but Susan did take something profound away from that incident. A psychiatrist at the hospital, after reviewing Sam's case history, pronounced that he had a particularly "malignant" form of bipolar disorder. He urged Susan to consider guardianship arrangements and residential placements.

But no one in that family was about to give up. Sam maintained a straight-A average throughout the return of his illness and the resumption of ECT; he was determined to be a neurologist, famous or not. And Susan thought he would get there, even if he took a nontraditional route. Although Sam was eager to go to the same college his brother attended, she suspected it might be better if he transitioned out of his small, "super-protective," private high school with a year or two of community college. But that decision could wait. When I caught up with Susan after Sam's second acute course of ECT, Sam was only a junior. He and his parents still had some time to consider their options.

In the meantime, Susan was just happy that Sam had finally moved back to his own bed after sleeping on a chaise in her room for two weeks, terrified someone would break into the house. Like the lab coat, it was a subtle sign, only this one was positive: an indication that Sam was improving. But there were lingering issues. Sam still struggled with anxiety. And although he had been an outgoing child, he no longer had any friends. "Sam would rather talk with adults about world hunger than gush about Justin Bieber with kids his own age," Susan told me, describing how he pursued his passion for science in college courses he took online. "This whole experience has aged him," she added sadly.

As it has aged her entire family. "Living with mental illness, living with a bright kid with so much potential who is completely debilitated—it's torturous," she said. When I pointed out that word had actually become a rallying cry for anti-ECT activists, she used it again: "The torture is living with the mental illness, not the ECT."

CHAPTER 9

Jonah, april 2010

MAINTENANCE BEGINS

APRIL 2, 2010

About 6:45, we head uptown for the last in Jonah's acute series of ECT. Liz isn't there, which saddens me, because I thought I'd have a chance to say goodbye and thank her for all her many kindnesses. The entire staff at Mount Sinai has been unbelievably warm, concerned, and accommodating. I think sometimes about the accusations levied against ECT doctors like Dr. Kellner by the anti-ECT movement—that they're just in it for the money. I find this hilarious on so many levels. I can just imagine a young Dr. Kellner consulting with upperclassmen about the specialty he should pursue. "If you really want the big bucks," one tells him, "forget about plastic surgery. Forget about radiology, anesthesiology, all the cushy jobs you've heard about. ECT is where the real money is. People will call you a Nazi and accuse you of torturing patients and violating their human rights, but it's totally worth the ostracization." Never mind common sense—there's actually good, hard data proving that ECT is a bargain compared to other forms of psychiatric treatment because it works so much faster: Canadian researchers analyzing inpatient admissions of adolescents with bipolar disorder found that those who received ECT rang up an average bill of $58,608 Canadian dollars, while those who refused it cost the hospital $143,264—almost two-and-a-half-times more.[1]

In her 2010 book *We've Got Issues*, Judith Warner examined why parents and psychiatrists give stimulants, antidepressants, and antipsychotics to young people. Although a common perception is that kids are medicated by greedy doctors and hyper-competitive parents worried about whether or not their average preschoolers will get into Harvard, Warner found after researching her book that wasn't the case: "Almost no parent takes the issue of psychiatric diagnosis lightly or rushes to 'drug' his or her child; and . . . responsible child psychiatrists don't either," she wrote.[2] And that's been my experience as well. All Jonah's psychiatrists—from Dr. Hetznecker to Dr. Wachtel to Dr. Kellner—have shown a tremendous commitment to Jonah's well-being. They've made themselves available to me on evenings and weekends, and have consulted with me so extensively by phone and email without charge that eventually I had to tell Dr. Hetznecker that I wanted him to bill me for his time. Despite all the failed medications, all the times I've despaired about ever being able to stop Jonah's aggression, his doctors have never given up, never ceased searching for the perfect solution. Is ECT the perfect solution? It's too early to say anything more than that it is helping for now. But regardless of whether it turns out to radically change Jonah's life or, like so many other interventions, ultimately stop helping, I will never doubt that Jonah's doctors recommended ECT because they believed it might be that perfect thing.

After our Liz-free ECT, Andy and I marshal a wobbly Jonah to the car and drive directly down to Atlantic City. It's Good Friday, so Andy has off, and we're taking the whole family down for the first shore weekend of the season. Marina will meet us with the rest of the kids plus the dogs. Even Oat and her husband Brendan are coming, just because they don't want to miss out on the fun. Jonah's aide, Amanda, will also be with us for part of the weekend, so we will be flush with help, which is good. The shore has been, in the past, a tough place for Jonah, and I'm wondering how the ECT-induced calm will hold up against the temptation of soft pretzels, French fries, churros, donuts, and so many other treats not even an arm's length away.

We're the first ones to reach the house, and after unloading the provisions we picked up at a Costco along the way, we call in an order for lunch for the whole gang at our favorite pizza place, Tony Baloney's (otherwise known in our household as "Eat Here," since a large sign, even bigger than the one saying "Tony Baloney's," with those words hung over the front door all last summer. Naturally, Jonah deduced the name of the restaurant must be "Eat Here.")

"I'd like to place an order for pick-up," I say.

"Go ahead."

"First, I'd like a hamburger, medium, with no bun, no cheese, no lettuce or tomato—nothing, just the patty," I begin.

"Is this for Jonah?" asks the voice on the other end that I don't recognize, but who clearly remembers us.

By the time Andy and Jonah have returned with two large pizzas, salads, wings, and Jonah's hamburger and French fries, everyone else has arrived. We devour our lunch, then Andy, Amanda, and Jonah head out on a walk so Andy can show Amanda the lay of the land. The rest of us clean up, get the kids ready, and about forty-five minutes later, we meet at a playground near the beach—one with a tennis court, so Andy and I can hit while the kids play. Jonah doesn't seem thrilled with the playground, but Amanda manages to keep him amused long enough for us to get a set in.

That night, we take advantage of our abundance of babysitters to meet an old college friend for dinner and poker at the Borgata. Day one of our long weekend, I think it's safe to say, is fun for everyone.

APRIL 3, 2010

Jonah sleeps until eight. This is such a departure for him—he's usually up by six thirty, but it can be much earlier—that instead of going for a run, as I was planning, I putter around the empty kitchen fretting: *Should I check on them? I don't want to wake them up. What if he's dead? He can't be dead. What if he's in a coma? Why is he sleeping so late?*

By the time Jonah does get up, get dressed, and eat breakfast, it's almost time to go pick up our boat, which has been stored at the dealership all winter. Jonah loves going on "fast boat rides," so I drop Jonah, Amanda, and Andy off at a ramp in Brigantine, where the dealer is waiting to put our boat in the water, then drive back to hang with the rest of the kids. I'm expecting Andy back in about half an hour when we will leave for Ocean City, since our favorite amusement pier, Castaway Cove, is opening for the season with its traditional Easter weekend ticket sale.

After the other kids are all dressed, I sit on the couch, facing the inlet, just relaxing and watching out for our boat with its distinctive orange canopy. After about forty minutes, Andy calls. "My navigation equipment isn't working right," he says. "I had a lot of trouble figuring out the bay. But I'll be back soon."

Another hour passes. I call Andy's cell phone, and Amanda answers. "Are you guys okay?" I ask.

"Yes, we're fine," she says. "I think we may be—." I hear Andy say something in the background. "Okay, no, we're not lost."

"Ask Andy if I should take the kids to Castaway Cove, and you guys can meet us when you get back," I say. "We're going to have to take two cars anyway."

I wait while Amanda repeats this to Andy; then, "He says no."

"Okay," I say, reclaiming my seat on the couch.

Finally, over two hours after I dropped them off, our boat pulls into the inlet. I run out to help them dock. "Was Jonah okay?" I ask Amanda, imagining how agitated Jonah might have grown as Andy fiddled with the controls, trying to figure out why his depth gauge was off, trying to remember everything he had learned about the boat last summer, our first summer as official boat people.

"He was great," Amanda says. "He had a smile on his face the whole time."

"Wow." I'm impressed. "Wasn't it freezing?"

Skinny Amanda, who never complains about anything, smiles. "Yes," she says. "It was."

Finally, we head out to Ocean City. Because of the ticket sale, as well as other Easter activities that are probably going on, traffic getting onto the island is brutal. Andy is somewhere ahead of me with Amanda and Jonah, Oat and Brendan have already gone home, and I have everyone else in my minivan.

"Can I play on your iPhone?" Gretchen asks. Erika has loaded all kinds of games onto my phone, including one I especially despise called "Ant Smasher," which makes the very realistic sound of a bug being squashed every time the kids press their thumbs against the virtual insects crawling across the screen. I guess I'm too disconnected from my inner child to understand why they find this so appealing.

"Not now," I say. "Daddy might try to call, and besides, I don't want to drain the battery."

"It's not fair," Gretchen whines. "Jonah always gets his iTouch in the car."

I know that experts believe parents should validate their children's feelings, even if they don't necessarily agree with them, and I do try, most of the time. I say, *Aaron, I understand you're upset that you lost rock, paper, scissors so now Gretchen gets the good light saber and you have to use the broken one, but you really shouldn't do rock, paper, scissors if you're not prepared to live with the results*, instead of what I really want to say, which is, *Don't be a sore loser*. But there is one thing I can't stand, which is hearing any of my children grumble because Jonah gets to watch his iTouch, or eat a plum instead of broccoli at dinner, or walk outside in bare feet. To be honest, they don't complain very often, but when they do, I shut it down immediately.

"Jonah needs his iTouch because he's autistic," I remind Gretchen. (When Erika was much younger, she used to tell people her brother needed certain accommodations because he was *artistic*, which I loved.) "You can chat with me or your brother or sisters, look through the American Girl catalogue, or play I Spy to pass the time. Jonah can't do any of that. His life is so much harder than yours—he'll never have friends, or get married, or have an interesting job, or see the world. Please don't ever let me hear you say that anything Jonah gets is unfair. It's what he'll never get that's really unfair."

Gretchen doesn't say anything—she's heard this spiel before. To validate her boredom at being stuck in traffic, I turn on the CD player and put on her favorite track, "I'm Being Swallowed by a Boa Constrictor."

Slowly, we inch forward. I crane my head fruitlessly, trying to spot Andy's pick-up truck, wondering how Jonah is doing. Sitting in traffic is another one of those things that has precipitated many frustrated outbursts, but—as I found out later—there were no problems. By the time we catch up with Andy, Amanda, and Jonah at Castaway Cove, Andy is most of the way through the enormous line. Amanda and Jonah have returned from the Ocean City Boardwalk where they had been dispatched to buy candy to occupy the kids while we wait for the tickets.

The weather report promised temperatures in the mid-sixties, but it never gets above fifty-four degrees that afternoon, according to the weather app on my iPhone. Marina and I are freezing as we escort Hilary and the twins from the carousel to the cars to the dragons—all their favorites. Andy and Amanda take Jonah and Erika on the big rides, including several turns on the Double Shot, the largest attraction on the pier. I'm sorry to miss the joy that erupts across Jonah's face the instant he and Erika shoot into the sky fast enough to suck the air from their lungs, even though I know I'll have plenty of opportunities to witness it over the course of the summer—we visit at least one of the Jersey shore amusement piers every time we go down to Atlantic City. All the kids love rides, but it's more than that for me. Jonah is, in general, a terrible big brother. He never hurt his younger brother or sisters, for which I'm profoundly grateful, but he's made it clear that he has little interest in them. Erika especially has tried over the years to engage him, to sing and draw for him the way I do, and has been met almost every time with an emphatic, "Erika, I'll be right back"—Jonah's unique, pronoun-challenged way of asking an individual to go away, presumably picked up after hearing me say so many times, "I'll be right back," before leaving his room to check Hilary's homework, find Aaron's shin guards, answer the phone, etc.

But at amusement parks, Jonah becomes the fearless big brother all younger siblings admire. Nothing is too high, too fast, too disorienting. He and Erika have gone on rides so insane they cost $25 because they practically launch you into orbit. When I watch them strap themselves into rides ominously named after natural disasters or bloodthirsty predators, all of Jonah's issues melt away, and I imagine how the two of them must appear to any casual bystanders: just another brother and sister, braving together centripetal forces that would turn their more timid parents inside out. And each time I stay on the ground, waving, I'm struck by this physical tolerance for extreme rides that Jonah and Erika share. It reminds me of other traits of Jonah's I attributed to his autism until I saw them echoed in my other kids, such as Hilary's precocious reading ability, or both Erika's and Aaron's tendencies to flap their hands when they get excited. This observation is always shadowed by my secret hope that my four younger children always appreciate how much they and Jonah have in common, even if his differences are so much more obvious.

Finally, at about five o'clock, Marina and I can take the cold no longer. Although Aaron sobs that he wants to stay, we arrange to meet Andy, Amanda, and Jonah for dinner back in Atlantic City. Jonah, Andy tells me, had a great time at the rides. He went on everything, instead of losing interest after one or two rides and perseverating on all the food everywhere, as he often did last summer. We end up at Eat Here again, when our first-choice restaurant informs us of its hour-long wait. After dinner, we drop off the kids and head out for another night with our friend at the Borgata. Amanda will leave after she puts Jonah to bed, so we want to take advantage of the help while we have it.

APRIL 4, 2010

Jonah doesn't sleep in again the next morning, but I'm already awake when he gets up at seven o'clock. In fact, I'm outside walking the dogs when I see Jonah come out through the front door. "Where do you think you're going?" I ask. Busted, Jonah follows me back upstairs, where I make him breakfast.

Jonah's elopement is still a tremendous problem. I'm not sure why I thought ECT might help with this also, but it hasn't. I guess it's helped a little bit—now, when Jonah's caught, he agreeably allows you to lead him back to wherever he's supposed to be, whereas before, diverting him from his object (usually food) often resulted in a tantrum. In fact, later, when we go to Steel Pier on the Atlantic City Boardwalk to take advantage of their ticket sale, Andy loses Jonah in the crowd. I had been following behind with Marina, Hilary, and the twins, since the three-year-olds are such slow walkers, while Andy, Jonah, and Erika went ahead, so I just leave the three younger kids with Marina and bolt through the Taj Mahal casino to Steel Pier as soon as I get Andy's frantic call. Almost immediately I run into Jonah, escorted by two security guards and holding a soft pretzel. Just like the time when Jonah managed to get his hands on a churro by himself, I'm impressed by his cunning; but just like that earlier time, I throw the pretzel away while he watches.

"If you stay with Mommy and Daddy the whole time we're at the rides, I'll get you a pretzel before we leave," I tell him. "But you have to stay with Mommy and Daddy. You cannot run away, and you can't just grab food!"

Andy appears even before I can call him to tell him I've got Jonah. He's tremendously relieved and immediately attempts to deduce from the shape of the pretzel which particular stand Jonah must have stolen it from, but even when he figures it out, the vendor refuses to accept his money—which immediately makes him my favorite pretzel vendor on the boardwalk. Few things touch me more than these small, generous moments with strangers—strangers who see how difficult it is to parent a child like Jonah and know they can't help in any global way, but decide they can let us step in front of them on line at the water slide, or stop and guide Jonah out of the busy road in front of our house the times he's escaped, or give him a free cinnamon roll when he steadfastly refuses to leave the convenience store without one (which, as expected, only increased Jonah's obsession with that little bodega; but hey, not everyone is an expert in behavior theory). In *The Boy in the Moon*, Ian Brown's memoir about his severely disabled son, he muses that Walker "has a purpose in our evolutionary project . . . he might be one (very small) step toward the *evolution* of a more varied and resilient ethical sense in a few members of the human species." It's nice to imagine Jonah this way, activating and maybe even enlarging the empathetic spirit in the random people who cross his path.

And I, since I *am* an expert in behavior theory, help this process along whenever I can with more tangible reinforcers than just our gratitude. After Jonah spends the rest of the evening at Steel Pier staying close by, following directions and being an overall good boy, he gets a pretzel and large lemonade from the same vendor—only this time, we pay for it.

APRIL 5, 2010

This morning, Erika and Hilary go back to school; the twins' break lasts one more day, but Jonah doesn't start again until Wednesday. It's a beautiful spring day, so I decide to do something I haven't done in a long time—take Jonah to the zoo, one of his favorite places, by myself. I consider taking Oat and the twins with us, but if there's anything harder than making a quick exit with an autistic eleven-year-old mid-tantrum, it's making a quick exit with an autistic eleven-year-old mid-tantrum and two three-and-a-half year olds who don't want to go home because they haven't had their camel rides yet! or had their faces painted! or seen the lions! In the end it seems easier to just take Jonah. Besides, it's an important moment, and I want him to have my undivided attention. If this is successful it opens up so many other opportunities—for me to take Jonah to the beach, or to Great Adventure, or even just to the mall on those days (and there are many every year) when he doesn't have school because the teachers have an in-service or just because his vacations don't completely align with those of the other kids.

After I send Erika and Hilary off to school, I take some time preparing Jonah for our outing. As much as he loves the zoo, it's also been the scene of some terrible rages: primarily, like many of his behaviors, over food. We always get lunch when we take the kids to the zoo; Jonah has come to expect his "ketchup and French fries" immediately upon arrival. Once, a few months before Jonah went to KKI, Andy and I took all the kids to the zoo, and since it was Labor Day Weekend, we got there shortly after it opened at nine thirty to beat the crowds. When we tried to explain to Jonah that he couldn't have ketchup and French fries at nine thirty, he had a huge tantrum—he went after Andy, then threw himself down on the concrete, screaming and thrashing. Once he calmed down, we "compromised" by having lunch at ten thirty.

This time, I decide to make a short list. After consulting with Jonah about what animals he wants to see, it looks like this:

1. Lions
2. Tigers
3. Bears
4. Ketchup and French fries
5. Tree house
6. Zebras
7. Go home

Because we won't be arriving at the zoo until after ten thirty and the snack bar will be open, I could just stack the odds in my favor by making ketchup and French fries first, but I'm putting my faith in ECT and testing him a bit. He doesn't even argue with me, and we take the list and get in the car.

It turns out that Number 1 should have been gas station. I'm perilously close to empty, so we stop at the station down the street from our house. Jonah recognizes a convenience store when he sees one, even if this particular gas station's idea of a mini mart consists of a few shelves of chips and Tastykakes, and one refrigerated case of drinks. "White chips," he says as I get back in the car after starting the pump, which is what he calls salt and vinegar potato chips because his favorite brand comes in a white bag.

"No chips," I tell him. "We're going to have ketchup and French fries at the zoo, remember?" He's sitting in the third row of my minivan, watching his iTouch, and he doesn't seem too upset by my answer.

After a few minutes, the pump stops, and I get out to replace the handle. I hear what sounds like the sliding door of my minivan, but when I jerk my head around, all I see is a couple getting into their car across the parking lot. I dismiss the sound as coming from them, get back into my car and head toward the zoo.

The entrance to the expressway that will take us into Philadelphia is just a mile or so down the road from the gas station, so in a couple of minutes I'm cruising at sixty-five miles an hour toward the zoo. "Hey Jonah, what animals are we going to see?" I call, inflecting my voice with the hyperbolic enthusiasm required to get Jonah's attention.

Jonah typically tunes out anything I say to him that doesn't include crucial words like "ketchup," so I'm not surprised when he doesn't answer.

"Jonah, what's Number 1?" I ask, so loud I'm almost yelling. This is what most of my conversations with Jonah look like: intense, repetitive effort on my part, followed at last by a word or phrase in reply. (Although, when properly incentivized, he's capable of lovely sentences. For example, once I scolded him after he tried to snatch a bite of my steak, "Jonah, we do not grab food off other people's plates! You need to ask me," and he replied, "Mommy, I want grab food off other people's plates. Please.") When Jonah was in preschool, I read that parents of language-delayed children should surround their kids with words, provide a constant soundtrack to their days by narrating everything they do or see. I think I managed to execute this strategy about as long as I followed the white-sugar-and-white-flour-free diet advocated in *What to Eat When You're Expecting*. Talking to someone who rarely talks back is very, very difficult. It's exhausting, frustrating, and ultimately, disheartening. I can only do it in bursts.

Silence. And then it strikes me: not only do I not hear Jonah, but I don't hear any songs or scraps of dialogue from his iTouch.

A sense of panic starts seeping through me, starting in my gut and spreading outward until I feel the chill in my teeth. I know what I will see when I shift my eyes to the rearview mirror to check out the back seat: nothing. The sound I heard at the gas station was my car door. In the twenty seconds my back was turned fitting the handle back into the pump, Jonah must have bolted from the car. And I'm stuck on the highway, heading in the opposite direction.

The sick feeling of knowing you've abandoned your child at the gas station is only slightly mitigated by the fact that Jonah's far less likely to dart into traffic or get into a stranger's car than he is to just wreak havoc in the convenience store. I imagine the scene:

Jonah opens a bag of chips and starts eating.
Attendant: Hey, kid! What are you doing?
Jonah grabs a bottle of Gatorade from the cooler.
Attendant: Hey, what's wrong with you? You have to pay
    for those!
Jonah happily eats chips and drinks Gatorade.
Attendant: Hey, Bob!! What's up with this kid here???

As I'm desperately trying to calculate how long it will take me to get back to the gas station, I realize that Marina may still be at the house. I call her cell and, thankfully, she is home and agrees to go pick up Jonah at the station and pay for whatever merchandise he's consumed. By the time I meet her there, Jonah is waiting in her car, still working on his bag of chips. "Marina, you can't reward him for this kind of behavior," I say, taking the chips away and throwing them in the trash can in front of Jonah. I hold on to the Gatorade, though—all those chips are bound to make him thirsty.

After this little incident, the rest of our outing is uneventful. When we get to the zoo, I direct Jonah's attention to our list. He doesn't even ask for ketchup and French fries until after we've wandered through Big Cat Falls, pressing our faces against the Plexiglas wall that separates us from a lion sprawled at our feet; looked unsuccessfully for Spectacled Bears in the Spectacled Bears exhibit; and satisfied our requirement for "Number 3 Bears" with the polar variety. The entire morning not only proceeds without any agitation at all, but it seems as if for the first time, Jonah is actually interested in the animals. He counts the tigers, then—when the zebra yard is perplexingly empty—leans his head on my shoulder while we watch the giraffes amble back and forth across their dusty pen.

After lunch, Jonah and I walk over to the little manmade pond to feed his discarded hamburger bun to the ducks. I know if I just hand him the roll, he'll chuck the whole thing into the water—which is, granted, the quickest and most efficient way of completing this task, if not exactly the point of it—so I tear the bread into little pieces, and he throws them. There are only two or three ducks in the water when we start, but once the birds mysteriously sense our activity, they come streaming from all sides of the pond: mallards; lumpy, mottled domestic ducks; and the aggressive Canadian geese that grab food right out of your hand. I know Jonah doesn't care about favoring the smaller, shyer ducks or avoiding the geese, but he humors me, waiting patiently for each scrap and tossing it where I direct him. I misquote one of Jonah's favorite lines from *Elmopalooza* to make him laugh. Instead of, "Grover, there are no penguins in New York City! Do you know what this means?" I say, "Jonah, there are no ducks in Philadelphia—" and although his eyes light up, and he grins in recognition, he interrupts me: "Stop singing."

"Everyone's a critic," I sigh in mock exasperation because I'm not exasperated at all. The birds keep coming, even though the hamburger bun is gone, and it's as if I can feel their life, energy, and hope flowing through us. The sun glints off the gold flecks in Jonah's hair and I lean over to plant a kiss on his head. He squirms away, saying, "No kiss." It's as typical a reaction as I would expect from an eleven-year-old boy, and it's so easy to believe we're done with the rages for good.

APRIL 7, 2010

I finally connect with Dr. Jaffe, Dr. Kellner's colleague at Belmont, and we schedule Jonah's first maintenance ECT for the next Monday. It will be ten days between treatments, but Dr. Jaffe tells us not to come on Friday, since he wants to be there for Jonah's first session and he's going to be out of town. I note the address of the hospital and hang up the phone, wondering if Jonah will be able to make it until Monday. He already seems more agitated today, although it's true he has a stomach virus and was sent home from school this morning after vomiting seven times. He's seemed fine since we got home, though—he asked for lunch and ate it with no signs of sickness. I wish, for about the millionth time, that I could peek inside Jonah's head to really understand what he's thinking and feeling. Does he still feel sick? Has the ECT worn off already? And why, for God's sake, does he punch himself in the nose when he's mad until his face is covered with blood?

APRIL 8, 2010

When Jonah grabs me by the back of my T-shirt, I'm utterly unable to free myself. Stupid, I scold myself as I try to twist away, but he is directly behind me and all I can do is flail while the collar of my shirt tightens around my neck. He's not really going to choke me, I know that—Amanda is right there, struggling to pry his fingers off my shirt. I can hear the fabric rip as he pulls harder. Before ECT I would never have turned my back on Jonah in the middle of a tantrum, but I had felt so secure that he wouldn't attack me that I sat down at the computer to type an email to Dr. Kellner and Dr. Wachtel while Jonah thrashed on the floor behind me. *Jonah's behavior has taken a serious nosedive in the past two days*, I wrote. I didn't get much farther than that before he went after me.

After Amanda helps pull Jonah off me, the two of us stand there while Jonah screams on the floor. We wait for him to sit calmly so Amanda can start the timer and Jonah can complete the one-minute time out procedure. But as many times as he takes a shuddering breath and says, "Yes," which he does when he wants her to start the timer, Jonah is completely unable to sit still for longer than a few seconds before he flops back on the floor, crying and pounding himself in the face. At first, I think all that's in store is a lot of crying like last night. That is, until he gets up and looks at me, and even as I say, "Jonah, you need to sit down," I know he's going to come after me again, and he does.

Matty is there instantly—I guess he was hovering outside the door of my office, waiting to see if he was needed. He quickly gets between Jonah and me, then directs Jonah back to the floor. Jonah hits Matty a few times before collapsing, and then Matty, Amanda, and I wait for Jonah to pull himself together.

And we wait.

For more than thirty minutes we wait. Later that night, when I come back to my email to Dr. Kellner and Dr. Wachtel, I write, *Honestly, I haven't seen him lose control like this in a long time—or rather, I haven't seen him suffer from such a complete inability to pull himself to-*

gether. And it's true. As intense as Jonah's behaviors have been before ECT, they were usually relatively short. Before we had the vocabulary to talk about Jonah's "rapid-cycling bipolar disorder," we would say, "Jonah doesn't hold a grudge." Five minutes after you disentangled his fingers from your hair, he'd be crawling in your lap for a hug.

After about twenty minutes, Matty squats down next to Jonah. "Take a deep breath," he says, modeling a loud exhale.

"Matty," I say.

He doesn't hear me. He tries again. "Deep breath, Jonah," he says, and Jonah manages one hiccupy inhale before trying to hit Matty on the head.

The time out procedure we use was designed by the behavior team at KKI and is straightforward and unambiguous. Jonah must sit for one minute without any behaviors; if behaviors do occur, the timer is stopped, reset for one minute, and only started once Jonah is sitting calmly. The plan also mandates as little attention as possible be directed toward Jonah during the time out. We're not supposed to even look at him until the minute is over, never mind talk to him, or try to soothe him. The logic is simple: you never want to reinforce negative behavior with positive attention. The last thing in the world we want Jonah to learn is that if he wants Mommy or Daddy or Uncle Matty to stop what we're doing and pay attention to him, all he has to do is attack someone.

I'm not sure if Matty doesn't know the details of the behavior plan, or if, at this moment, he doesn't care. I can't really blame him. Jonah is screaming with a primal distress he seems completely incapable of bearing, his suffering is so acute—and why? What provoked this tantrum? Absolutely nothing. Jonah was up to "choice" on his schedule of activities, which means that no demands were being placed on him. He had free access to his iTouch, YouTube, and his markers. This tantrum was due solely to some kind of disruption within his brain. Of course, we all just want to help him. But when Matty puts his hand on Jonah's head and tries to stroke his hair, I step forward. "Matty," I say again, and he stands up.

Finally, Jonah makes it through his one minute. Since he wet himself during his rage, Amanda and I guide him to the bathroom and I help him through a quick shower. Then Amanda assists him with his pajamas while I get his medicine. I lie down with him for a few minutes, and he immediately falls asleep. I'm not surprised he's drained after that extensive a fit.

When I get back to my computer I finish my email: *Dr. Kellner, if you get this message tonight, let me know if you have an opening tomorrow morning and I'll drive him up to Mount Sinai, because I'm not sure he's going to make it through the weekend like this.* Although Jonah has an appointment for his first maintenance ECT at Belmont on Monday, it seems impossibly far away—especially because Jonah is supposed to go to Camp Joy for his second and last respite weekend of the season. It's hard to imagine the camp director not calling us to come get Jonah if he has another fit like the one he had tonight. And we're supposed to take the other kids to visit a friend in Greenwich who was recently diagnosed with cancer. Should we cancel our trip? I wonder. Should we cancel Jonah's weekend at Camp Joy? Most importantly, I wonder how Jonah could have tumbled so far, so fast. After the acute course of ECT, I thought he would be able to go a week or more between treatments. I stare at my computer screen, hoping to find an instant response from Dr. Kellner. But it's almost nine o'clock; as far as I know, he might be asleep already. ECT starts at seven in the morning. Who knows how early he has to get up?

The phone rings; it's Andy, calling from New York where he went for a firm bowling party. I spill out everything that happened. I can hear the sounds of the city in the background and know that Andy is distracted by the need to find a cab and get to Penn Station for the eleven p.m. train home, but I don't want him to hang up.

Just then, my iPhone, which I dropped next to me when I collapsed into bed, pings. It's an email from Liz: "Dr. Kellner just called and asked me to contact you regarding your request to bring Jonah in for ECT tomorrow. Please come on up."

Immediately I feel both a rush of relief and despair: relief, because Jonah won't have three more days of such profound suffering; and despair, because this means that I will miss something Aaron has been looking forward to all year—tomorrow he will serve as Shabbat King of his pre-school class.

In retrospect, I know this won't seem like a big deal—it's not like I'm missing his high school graduation. Aaron will get to carry his class' tzedekkah can to the front of the sanctuary and shake the coins into the big school jug. He'll get to come up to the bima with the other Shabbat Kings and Queens from the other classes and help the rabbi say the blessing. He'll get to march down the aisles carrying a stuffed torah. But for three-year-old Aaron, it's a tremendous deal, one he's been anticipating since October, when Gretchen was Shabbat Queen and everyone came—me, Andy, Marina, Oat, Aunt Keri, Molly—to read a story and take pictures and share treats. All winter he had asked, "When will I be Shabbat King?" and I had said, "In the spring." After that, whenever the sun was shining, the temperatures were unseasonably warm, or even if anyone even uttered the word "spring," Aaron would say, "Am I going to be Shabbat King?"

Finally, I am sobbing. All the tears I tried (only semi-successfully) to hold back during Jonah's tantrum so Matty and Amanda wouldn't see how upset I was came flooding out. I tried to explain to Andy everything he would need to do to make Aaron's day special without me. "Aaron wants to bring donuts, so don't forget to stop at Dunkin' Donuts for munchkins on the way to school," I say. "And I bought a book about a bear in underwear to read to the class, you know how much he loves bears—"

Andy interrupts me, "Should I take Jonah tomorrow?"

I pause. Of course, this is what I want—to be there for Aaron, to see the excitement and pride on his little face. But I know Andy wants to be there, too. Whenever we split up as a family, particularly on the weekends, Andy goes with Jonah, because he is the only one who can really manage him when he is in a full-fledged rage. They spend so much time together—shopping, hiking, going to the rock-wall gym or the water park—that Andy has told me several times he feels he doesn't know the twins very well. This is a great opportunity for him to share a special day with Aaron. Besides, he won't be home until after one in the morning. It seems insane, and probably unsafe, to ask him to get up at four thirty to drive to Mount Sinai.

"I'll go," I say.

APRIL 9, 2010

When I grab my phone to throw in the car for the drive up to Mount Sinai, I see an email from Dr. Wachtel. She answered my email at 11:13 last night: *As Charlie* [Charles Kellner] *knows, my pa-*

tients have all defied classic maintenance paradigms for ECT, with most requiring very, very slow weaning in ECT frequency from thrice weekly, to twice weekly (for several weeks), to then alternating 2/1/2/1, then to once weekly, then maybe to q9 days, and maybe to q14 days, if I'm lucky. I've been burned many times trying to wean then getting a call from a mom that her child is stuporous, rigid, cold, can't eat and can't pee. WHY these autistic kids need such intense schedules of ECT is on the top of my list of questions to answer. Her words are reassuring on so many levels. First, it just warms me that both she and Dr. Kellner—who is apparently holed up somewhere in Nowheresville, South Carolina, this week (which is why he couldn't call me himself but had to ask Liz to do it)—answered my plea for help immediately. Just knowing they are there for me whenever I need them makes me feel so much less alone. It's hard to imagine we won't figure this thing out with two such brilliant minds working together, combining forces to save my son.

But Dr. Wachtel's email calms me even more because it's clear that she wouldn't have expected Jonah to last a week at this point in his treatment. What seemed last night to be catastrophic, a sure sign that ECT was not the miracle we had hoped—no, we had *needed* it to be—seems now, in the slowly dawning light of a new day, to just be another minor obstacle in Jonah's path to recovery. Yes, it stinks that Jonah is still suffering so profoundly; and yes, it stinks that I have to miss Aaron as Shabbat King. But after a night's sleep, even one as abbreviated as mine was last night, it seems easier to focus on the big picture.

Jonah's ECT goes smoothly, and we are on our way home when my friend calls to cancel our trip to Greenwich. When I tell Andy, he is clearly not too disappointed. Although we both wanted to cheer up our friend, and opportunities for us to travel with the kids are limited since we hesitate to take Jonah to homes that have not been appropriately "Jonah-proofed" (as our friend's immaculate Greenwich mansion clearly has not been), he admits he was dreading the drive. And although it seems a waste of a Camp Joy weekend not to go away or at least do something we can't really do with Jonah, in the end we decide that just relaxing at home is taking advantage enough. After an uneventful afternoon and evening, during which Jonah is much happier, Amanda takes him to Camp Joy, and we take Erika, Hilary, and Gretchen to see *How to Train Your Dragon*. Of course we wanted to take Aaron too, but the Shabbat King was so exhausted from his day of festivities that he fell asleep at five o'clock and slept through until the next day.

APRIL 12, 2010

Since Dr. Wachtel and Dr. Kellner both agree that Jonah isn't ready to taper down to one treatment a week, I keep the appointment I had scheduled for Jonah's first maintenance ECT at Belmont for Monday morning. It's such a pleasure to drive only fifteen minutes to ECT instead of two hours. I leave at seven o'clock, fully expecting to have time to drop Jonah off at school, then come back to the house for a cup of coffee before changing and heading out to a tennis match I have at eleven

I guess I'm used to Mount Sinai where Liz never made us wait. But the Mount Sinai ECT team had access to a PACU with eleven beds; the Belmont unit has three beds, and Jonah is scheduled to be the fifth patient. This means we wait more than an hour. I make a mental note to arrive by six thirty on Friday when we're next scheduled for a treatment, so Jonah can be one of the first ones in. Still, he is very good, watching his iTouch and consulting with his list. He asks if he can kick off his crocs to spin, and I tell him sure. Meanwhile, I watch a group of inpatients in hospital pajamas who have been shepherded up to a lab adjoining the ECT suite to have their blood drawn. I wonder what it is that has brought them here. They all appear fine—one is chatting about the credits she needs to complete her high school degree. As they file back toward the elevator, another young woman says goodbye to Jonah and holds up her hand for a high-five, which he ignores.

Finally, it's Jonah's turn. They have him knocked out in just a few minutes, and I wait outside for the treatment to be over. When the nurse's aide invites me back in, he's still sleeping. I had told Dr. Jaffe that at Mount Sinai, Jonah was given a dose of Versed to make sure he slept long enough to have his vitals taken because the first time he had ECT, he woke up agitated and tried to pull off his oxygen tube and blood pressure cuff before the staff was satisfied his signs were stable. Dr. Jaffe tells me they don't have Versed at Belmont, but that they gave him Ativan—which, he tells me, is similar. When the nurse offers me a chair, I decline. At Mount Sinai it was probably about five minutes between when Liz called us back to Jonah's bedside to when he was up and ready to walk out the door.

Five minutes pass. Fifteen, then thirty. Jonah doesn't wake up. Three pretty nursing students hover over him, calling his name, but he doesn't respond at all. The nurse anesthetist checks his oxygenation and pulse. Everything is fine, but he's out cold. Dr. Jaffe comes to check on him, wondering whether his Ativan dose was too high. We discuss skipping the Ativan altogether next time, since they also use a different anesthetic at Belmont, one that lasts about twenty minutes, as opposed to the extremely short-acting agent they use at Mount Sinai.

Still, Jonah sleeps. Nick, his teacher, texts me to ask when Jonah is coming to school. I text him back, saying that I don't know if he's going to make it at all. Anxiously, I watch the clock. Worrying about something as bourgeois as tennis always seems so shallow to me, but the fact is that three other people are going to be waiting at a tennis court at eleven, and if I don't show up, they won't have much of a match. No one likes playing "Canadian,"—two against one—and it's much too late to get in touch with all three of them to reschedule.

I step outside to call Marina. Fortunately, she's home. She agrees to come meet me at Belmont with my tennis stuff and to take Jonah back home to sleep off the Ativan. Naturally, I don't tell Dr. Jaffe or the nurses what my appointment is. I understand it's not the most sympathetic excuse in the world. And I certainly wouldn't have left Jonah to go running or take a spin class, something that doesn't involve a commitment to other people. I also would have broken that commitment in an instant if Jonah really needed me, but Dr. Jaffe is clear: Jonah's sleeping because he got too much Ativan. He's not in any danger. As soon as he's even the slightest bit responsive we can take him home and let him rest there.

And that is what we do. Marina meets me at Belmont, and as soon as Jonah is able to mutter "yes" when one of the nursing students asks, "Are you excited about your pretzel and lemonade?" we help him into a wheel chair and wheel him down to the car. I tell Marina that if Jonah perks up in the next hour, she can drive him to school. But what actually happens is that Jonah gets home, collapses into bed, and sleeps until noon.

Later that night, Jonah is very agitated with one of his aides, Candace. But as much as he cries, he's not aggressive with her. It's always hard to know what provokes these moods, but given what he's been through today, it could easily be Ativan-induced fatigue. I decide not to worry too much about it, for now.

APRIL 22, 2010

We've gotten into a routine at Belmont: on Mondays and Fridays, either Marina or I wake Jonah a little after six o'clock so we can be through registration and waiting in the ECT lounge by six-thirty. There are only three beds in the ECT unit, and there might be six to ten outpatients waiting for a turn by the time the doors open at seven, so we've learned to get there early. After the first day, Jonah hasn't been given any Ativan at all, and he's alert and ready to go to school by ten o'clock.

And he's been doing so well, both at home and at school. This afternoon, Nick Boss leaves me the following voicemail: "Hi, Amy, how are you doing, it's Nick. I'm just calling to let you know—I know you've seen the data sheets, but I just wanted to let you know before you go to the doctor that this week has been really great. No behaviors, excellent, very happy, very attentive and responsive—it seems that we've reached a therapeutic level all around, between what we're doing, and the ECT, everything. I'm just very happy. Great week."

I smile and play the message again. Nick is one of the most laid back, laconic people I've ever met. I've never, in the sixteen months he's worked with Jonah, ever heard him gush.

CHAPTER 10
Alex

I knew, intellectually, that ECT didn't work for everybody. I knew it wasn't a magic bullet, a miracle—even if I may have used those words in private conversations to describe Jonah's transformation. But I don't think I really believed it until ECT failed to help a young man whose mother had pursued it on my recommendation.

Lisa had first emailed me in June 2011 about her autistic son Alex, then thirteen. Two of the members of Alex's home team also worked at Milagre, Jonah's school, and had reported back to her how effective ECT was in ameliorating the aggressive behaviors that Lisa was finding increasingly difficult to control in Alex. After we spoke on the phone, she explored the possibility of taking Alex to Mount Sinai, but the bureaucratic hurdles seemed insurmountable. Plus, she had just committed $1,200 a month for a renowned behavior analyst. She decided she might as well give the analyst a chance.

Sixteen months later, Alex was worse than ever. Although Lisa was impressed with the knowledge and commitment of the analyst, in retrospect she understood this effort was doomed to fail. Behavioral interventions work best on behaviors with clear environmental triggers—such as demands from parents or teachers, or denied access to favorite toys, foods, or activities. Alex's behaviors—like Jonah's— were unpredictable, occurring under any and all circumstances, even during his favorite activities, like jumping on the trampoline with his brothers. These intrinsically motivated behaviors are caused by neuropsychiatric disturbances, not environmental factors, and generally require medical treatment. Although the analyst was able to teach the family coping strategies that were somewhat effective in reducing the frequency of Alex's episodes, his increasing size and the resulting increase in intensity made them almost impossible to manage. By that point, Lisa and her husband, Jack, had set up a padded area in their house in a desperate attempt to contain their son's rages. But he was so big and strong, Lisa couldn't get him there safely on her own. In September 2012, Alex attacked her in her closet; Kevin, the oldest of her four sons, came running to find his mother on the floor with Alex on top of her. Her youngest son, Drew, had already locked himself in their addition, following the emergency plan Lisa and Jack had designed to keep their ten-year-old safe. "I've got this!" Lisa called to Kevin, because she couldn't let Alex know she was losing the ability to handle him.

But she didn't have it. By the time Kevin pulled Alex off her, she had lost such a huge hunk of hair that she later had to get a very short cut to hide the bald spot. More painfully, Alex had dislocated her thumb. Lisa, who was a nurse before Alex's need for constant supervision necessitated she give up her job, snapped it back in herself. She was afraid the doctors at the ER where she and Kevin drove Alex as soon as they could wrestle him into their van would commit him if they knew. She would let them medicate him, calm him down. But she wouldn't let them institutionalize him.

It was clear at this point that ECT was her best chance to keep that from happening. I introduced her to Dr. Jaffe, who agreed to treat Alex at Belmont. In the weeks between Alex's ER visit and his first ECT, Lisa's certainty that ECT would help after everything else had failed was the only thing that kept her going. "I had Jack convinced ECT was the answer to everything," she told me. "We had no idea how we would pay for it. If insurance didn't pay, we were prepared to sell our house, that's how sure I was it was going to work. ECT worked for 80 percent of people, according to my research. We put all our eggs in the ECT basket. There was no back up."

———————

Lisa's vigilance is older than Alex himself; she hemorrhaged during the third month of her third pregnancy and was told her fetus only had a 20 percent chance of survival. Given her medical background, she expected this trauma might result in developmental delay. "I told my mom I could handle anything as long as he wasn't autistic," she remembered, smiling at the irony. "I pictured the kids I knew when I was young that were autistic. They were non-verbal, stimmy—I assumed they had no interest in the world."

Alex wasn't like that at all. As a baby, he was happy, engaged, with good eye contact. Still, Lisa knew something was wrong. He was floppy, with poor muscle tone. Then he failed to meet early milestones. When he was seven months old, Alex was diagnosed with mild cerebral palsy and developmental delay. Lisa was ready. By the time he was one year old, he was already getting occupational, physical, and speech therapy. She engaged a Special Ed teacher to come to the house to supplement the therapies he was getting through her county's Early Intervention unit.

All this effort seemed to help. Alex developed a lot of language, even if it was a bit truncated compared to the lush sentences her older sons had spoken as toddlers. He was very social, seeking out his brothers to play tag and jump with him on the trampoline. But new problems appeared as he grew older. By the time he started a special pre-school, Alex was unfocused and hyper. Teachers suggested that Lisa take him to a developmental pediatrician for evaluation, which she initially resisted. "I felt he had all the services he needed at home," she told me. "And I didn't want him to be labeled." It took six months before she decided to get Alex evaluated and another six months to get an appointment. Alex was five years old when he was finally diagnosed with pervasive development disorder not otherwise specified (PDD-NOS), a milder form of autism, and ADHD.

"It was during the evaluation that I first saw really disruptive behaviors," Lisa told me. "Alex was throwing stuff in the trash can, ignoring the doctor. He would only behave well if he had one-on-one adult attention."

That kind of attention was increasingly difficult for Alex to get, since Drew had just been born. Alex was very aggressive toward his new brother, knocking over his bassinet, then pushing or tripping him once he started walking. Punishments had little effect because Alex seemed to enjoy negative as much as positive attention; he would tell his mother, "Put me in time out." Lisa's solution was to coax and encourage him, and heavily reinforce good behavior— which basically amounted to "a lot of bribing." Regardless of how she responded to Alex one thing was clear: he needed to be constantly supervised. "Drew has never had two parents," she said. "One of us has always been with him, while the other was with Alex." Kevin and Brian, the second-oldest son, were called upon to watch Alex if the assigned parent had to run to the bathroom or take a phone call. The family was too afraid he might hurt the baby, throw the remote control in the fish tank, or start ripping up whatever papers he could get his hands on to ever leave him alone.

School didn't help at all. Lisa was home schooling her two older sons, but decided to enroll Alex in a Verbal Behavior (VB) class for autistic children run by her local Intermediate Unit. She was such a huge believer in the precepts of VB—which emphasizes shaping language in the natural environment—that Alex had received twenty hours/week of VB therapy at home for the previous two years. Lisa had even gone to trainings herself so she could in turn teach the aides provided by the county.

But this class was, as the hosting school nicknamed it, a "zoo." The kids, mostly lower-functioning than Alex, were constantly screaming and escaping into the hallway. Alex hated it so much he had to be forced on the bus every morning. Lisa worked continuously with his teachers on strategies to help Alex succeed. She and Jack reluctantly agreed to try giving their son stimulants for his ADHD, but Ritalin made him even more hyper and Strattera made him moody and tearful. Then came the day in second grade when Alex came home with finger-shaped bruises and cuts from fingernails under his arms. He told his mother the teacher had hurt him. Lisa pulled him out of school immediately. From that day on, Alex was home schooled with his brothers.

The end of school seemed like a good opportunity for Lisa to really commit to stabilizing Alex biomedically. She found a doctor two states away that followed the Defeat Autism Now (DAN) protocol, which prescribes treatments designed to redress the toxin levels and immune deficiencies that some alternative practitioners believe cause autism. Over the next two years, she and Jack spent more than $40,000 on IV chelation, antivirals, a full Lyme panel, hyperbaric oxygen treatment, antibiotics for PANDAS, supplements, anti-inflammatories, and low-dose naltrexone. Jack, an automotive front-end specialist, was working seventy hours a week to pay for it all. When Alex's behaviors failed to improve after all these interventions, the DAN doctor advised Lisa to consult a psychiatrist—which is kind of like a Toyota salesman sending a customer to a Ford dealership. Lisa was devastated. "That was one of my lowest moments," she said.

Alex's adventures in psychopharmacology—which are still ongoing—have been similarly frustrating. Beginning in fourth grade, he has been prescribed Geodon, lithium, Abilify, Depakote, Lamictal, Ativan, and countless other drugs that typically caused activating effects completely opposite the stabilization his parents were desperately seeking. The benzodiazepine Klonopin caused Alex to have a psychotic break during which he hid in the basement for four days, ranting about hurting people, running upstairs to use the bathroom, then immediately retreating. Later, when Alex was twelve, the psychiatrist prescribed the antipsychotic Seroquel. Low-dose antipsychotics had successfully taken the edge off Alex's rages in the past, but higher doses had made him anxious. This time, the psychiatrist insisted on pushing the dose to therapeutic levels. "Alex shoved Drew down the stairs," Lisa told me. "When I called the psychiatrist, she increased the dose again. Drew was sleeping on the floor of our room, we were so afraid Alex would wake up in the middle of the night and hurt him." After the second increase, Alex locked himself in his room and went "berserk," according to Lisa. "He smashed the walls with his TV and put his head through the wall hard enough to bend the beam." Lisa called 911. By the time the police arrived, Alex had calmed down. Still, the officers wanted to take him to the ER. Lisa allowed it, not understanding that patients brought into the ER by police following 911 calls in her county can't be taken home unless the doctor permits it. And this doctor threatened to sign a 302 commitment order unless Lisa voluntarily admitted her son to a psych ward.

Lisa spent eighteen panicked hours in the ER, trying to convince doctors that Alex didn't need to be hospitalized, explaining over and over that his rage was due to a medication reaction. In the end, a friend arrived and threatened to sue the hospital for failing to provide appropriate medical treatment unless Alex was immediately released—despite the fact that he had bashed his head through a wall, he had never been given a CT scan or checked for head injuries. The ploy worked; Lisa and Alex were free to go home.

But go home to what? Alex had just hit puberty. His testosterone tripled seemingly overnight, and over the course of that year he grew four inches. Diagnosed with bipolar disorder in 2011, his mood swings became more pronounced. He began saying terrifying things like, "If Drew got hit by a car, would he die?" and "If Drew got hurt, would you be sad?" Every wall in their house was studded with holes where Alex had put his feet, hands, or head through them. He stuffed anything he could find down the toilets—including expensive electronics—so there were days when there was no place to go to the bathroom because every toilet was clogged. It got to the point where the bathroom doors were kept locked and the cats—one of which Alex had thrown down the basement steps—were kept locked in the addition and everyone in the family was afraid all the time that someone would forget, leave a door open, and Alex would do something horrible.

Nights were no better. When Alex was in a manic state his sleep was very erratic. Melatonin and other natural sleep remedies had no effect on him. Despite Lisa's fear that he might hurt his younger brother or inflict more damage on their already battered house—like the time he got up at four in the morning to fling the contents of the litter boxes around the basement, a noxious mess it took two days to clean up—she didn't dare lock him in at night. She had a friend whose autistic ten-year-old daughter had jumped out her bedroom window and broken both legs after being locked in her room at night. Instead, Lisa slept on the floor outside his room in a sleeping bag.

"I just kept going. I had no other option," Lisa said. "My family has since told me that I was crazed, that they wanted me to stop. I think I would have gotten divorced rather than stop, if that's what my husband told me to do."

Keep in mind that throughout this period, Lisa was homeschooling her three oldest boys. She had reluctantly enrolled Drew in a local Christian school when he was in second grade. "It wasn't optional," she explained to me. "It was out of control here, Drew couldn't be home." Still, for six hours a day, she took Kevin, Brian, and Alex to home schooling co-ops, playgrounds, and museums. Alex always came, even to Kevin's baseball games and wrestling matches. Outside of school hours, Lisa worked with her church to set up reverse inclusion opportunities for Alex and other kids with disabilities to spend time with typical peers. "I really felt that if I kept Alex immersed in the community, he would be OK," Lisa said. But no one was OK—not Alex, whose weekly fits were increasing in both frequency and intensity; not Kevin, who had anxiety attacks when he was out with friends because he was afraid of what was happening at home; not Brian, who spent all his time holed up in his room; not Drew, who still has a scar on the back of his head where Alex clubbed him with a dog bone; and not Lisa and Jack, who were both on blood pressure medication because of the unremitting stress. Said Lisa, "We were living on the edge."

Alex finally got his first ECT the day before his fifteenth birthday. Although Jack was concerned about any discomfort Alex might experience, Kevin shared his mother's unqualified optimism. He had taken a psychology class in college, where he was studying to be an occupational therapist, that had described ECT very positively, so he had no negative stereotypes. "At this point, we were desperate," he told me. "So it didn't seem to me like a cruel idea at all." And his hopes were very reasonable; he knew that even if ECT stopped Alex's behaviors, he would still be autistic. "Alex running around hooting, flapping—I would love that," he said, imagining a different, happier kind of chaos returning to their house, like the times when Alex would insist on buying clown noses or stuffed clowns or clown masks when he saw them in stores because Lisa had told him once that Kevin was terrified of clowns when he was a baby, and Alex loved to chase his brother around the house with his purchases, trying to scare him.

Alex was put on the standard acute course of three treatments a week, and although ECT left him sleepy, otherwise he appeared to be handling it well. He complained of mild headaches, which responded to Toradol and ibuprofen. There were no obvious cognitive issues, which was what Lisa was most concerned about. Alex's recall was good during intensive teaching time (ITT), when his aides worked with him on everything from conversation skills—such as asking and answering WH questions (starting with what, when, where or why) and talking about things that weren't present—to practical tasks, like hand washing and typing. During that first week, he had no behaviors, but Lisa didn't want to get her hopes up. Alex's behaviors were always episodic: intense rages followed by days of peace. She couldn't rule out the possibility he was just having a good week.

A snowstorm canceled Alex's first treatment of the following week. The next appointment proceeded as scheduled, but by the fifth ECT, "it was like the devil had reared his head," Lisa said. Alex came out of anesthesia with the agitation and pressured speech symptomatic of mania. Like Sam, he was one of the less than five percent of bipolar patients whose ECT triggers a manic episode. By the seventh treatment, Alex was attacking his mother as soon as he regained consciousness. Dr. Jaffe gave him Ativan to calm him down, but as with virtually everything else Alex has been prescribed, it had the opposite effect. After a few doses, Alex was psychotic, attacking his brothers and parents and destroying the house. An IV dose of Ativan administered after his ninth ECT sent Alex into a psychotic rage that lasted twenty-four hours and required four people—Lisa, Brian, Jack, and Jack's twin brother—to manage.

At this point, Lisa and the Belmont team were just trying to get Alex the fifteen treatments he would need before Dr. Jaffe could say for sure whether he was a non-responder. Dr. Jaffe stretched out the treatments a bit, dropping to twice a week, hoping Alex would tolerate them better. Alex was still activated, but the first two were more bearable. Then, after the third, Alex attacked Lisa and Brian for almost an hour. He hurled a full bottle of cleaner at the stove, denting it; upended the table; and threw the TV through a wall. Lisa and Brian desperately tried to defend themselves with big football blocking pads while trying to guide Alex to the padded area, which had since grown to take over the entire living room—the walls and floors of which were now lined with mattresses, the windows boarded and covered with foam. But Alex was just too strong for them.

Lisa and I were having coffee in a Starbucks when she told me this story, comparing notes about our own experiences and those of other families we knew. She said there was one thing we all had in common. "We're all living in the unacceptable, but getting by. But everyone has a breaking point, where they're not getting by any more." That day was in November 2012, when Alex's rage left his seventeen-year-old brother shaking and crying on the floor because he could no longer protect his mother. "That was my breaking point," Lisa said. The next day, Alex was admitted to a specialized inpatient unit for autistic kids with dangerous behaviors where he spent two months. "It crushed me," she said. "I had fought against this with everything I had."

In theory, this unit should have been the perfect place to finally find the answers to Alex's unpredictable rages and bizarre medication reactions. Staff members were purportedly experienced working with this population, so at the very least they should have been able to keep Alex and those around him safe. And the doctors supported the use of ECT, agreeing to transport him back and forth to Belmont to finish his acute course of treatment.

But the reality was much different. Alex's condition rapidly deteriorated. He completed the acute course of ECT with no improvement. When Dr. Wachtel, who was consulted on his case, advised that Alex may be one of a few patients who would benefit from the atypical antipsychotic Clozaril alone, or in conjunction with ECT, the doctors on the unit balked—just as I did when Dr. Kolevzon suggested Clozaril for Jonah during our appointment at Mount Sinai before his first ECT—because of its potentially fatal side effects. Instead, the unit doctors followed a haphazard medication strategy Lisa dismissed as a "med party," in which old medications were abruptly discontinued without a weaning period, new ones were introduced, and aggression was met with both physical and chemical restraint in the form of emergency sedatives that inevitably made Alex more agitated, not less. His behaviors quadruped over the course of his stay, including an increase in self-injury that left his ear red and swollen and his arms covered with bloody scratches.

Not all his wounds were self-administered. Alex was bitten and pinched by other patients; one twisted his genitals so hard he still had bruises a month later. Although Lisa was informed that her son had been grabbed, the location of the injury wasn't initially disclosed. The hospital also wasn't forthcoming about the psychological abuse Alex received; one young man would continuously tell Alex to hit himself in the head until he would get so agitated he would do it—which then, perversely caused Alex to be punished. He lost twenty pounds because he was so afraid of the other patients that he couldn't tolerate the dining room. When Lisa visited him, as she did every day, he ran to her and cried, "This is a nightmare!" But Lisa didn't find out how much of a nightmare it was until the end of his admission, when she finally demanded to see his entire medical record.

In January 2013, Alex was discharged after making "little to no progress," according to the hospital's own records. He was transferred to a residential treatment facility (RTF) that Lisa begged to accept him even though he was still unstable and required restraint several times a day. She just had to get him out of the hospital. "I was so excited and relieved when they said they would take him," Lisa told me. "I thought that things couldn't possibly get any worse, which meant they had to get better."

But things didn't get better. Although the RTF tried to work with Alex, he was just too traumatized from his hospitalization. "What it turned into was Alex staying in his room twenty-three hours a day," Lisa said. "He never wanted to come out. He wouldn't talk to the staff—if they talked to him, he would scream at them. If other kids made noise, even happy noises, he screamed. There wasn't a lot of aggression, but he couldn't pair with the staff or the other kids." And the regression that started in the hospital continued. After a month at the RTF, Alex could no longer hold a conversation. He refused to shower and began wiping his face on his sleeve during meals because there were no napkins on the tables.

The RTF's solution to Alex's rages was to keep adding different medications, despite the fact that this strategy had failed so miserably at the hospital. Alex ended up on five different drugs, the combination of which gave him a seratonin toxicity that left him so imbalanced he could barely walk. "We were at a crossroads," Lisa told me. "If we kept him there, it meant a life of institutionalization— heavily medicated, terrified, he wouldn't have gotten better. And I wasn't OK. I don't know what a nervous breakdown looks like, but I was heading for one." The final straw came one February night after Lisa had spent all day at the RTF. Alex had passed the previous night in the ER after bashing his head against the wall, and she could tell it calmed him to have her with him. "Alex didn't need any restraints while I was there, but at eight o'clock, when I got ready to leave, they wanted me to walk him to the restraint room where four men were ready, anticipating a major blow-up after I left. I said, 'Alex, get your shoes and jacket, we're going home.' And we walked right out."

Yanking Alex out of the RTF was an impulsive decision that Lisa readily admitted her family wasn't ready for. She brought him home to a construction zone. Jack was trying, in Alex's absence, to repair all the holes in the walls, while ultimately redesigning the house to accommodate both Alex's needs and those of his other sons. By the time I visited the family in March, Jack had built an "in-law suite" with its own separate entrance, so Brian and Drew could watch TV or do their homework, insulated from Alex's vacillating behaviors. Lisa had weaned Alex down to two medications; he had recovered his balance and was back to playing basketball and jumping on the trampoline. Slowly, Alex was recovering from the combined trauma of the hospital and the RTF. "When he got home, it was horrible," Lisa told me. "Alex had lost so many skills. He couldn't get his own food. He was afraid of plates and glasses, because he had eaten on paper plates for so long, he was afraid he would break them. He was afraid of the bathroom, of the dark, of going to bed. We had to put a mattress on the floor of his room, and Jack or I had to sleep with him. It was like having a baby again." But she had no regrets. "Even if I'm woken up six times during the night, I know Alex is in his bed, he's safe, no one is hurting him."

Alex was having a good day when I saw him. He had just come back from a bowling outing with his aide where he scored, he told us, two strikes. He was very conversational, although he speaks so quickly that at times it was hard for me to understand him. "Where's Jonah?" he wanted to know. "Is he autistic?" He asked about Aaron and Andy, but had no interest in hearing about Erika, Hilary, or Gretchen. His overall preoccupation with patrilineage was evident when the conversation turned to Barack Obama, whom Alex knew was president, even if he was more concerned with the fact that Obama had two daughters, but no sons.

I had brought Alex a stack of old *Entertainment Weekly* magazines, since I knew he liked to rip out pictures of celebrities, cute babies, pretty girls. Some he would laminate; others he would tuck into his treasured trucks and carom them around the basement. Lisa and I left Alex and Jack with the magazines and went out to dinner. It was the first time Lisa had been out of the house all week. Although she has some support staff, the bulk of Alex's care falls on her. "I gave up everything—my disability ministry at the church, my running," she said, adding that she had been training for a half-marathon. "I'm just backing off everything that requires planning or commitment."

Lisa must have read the sympathy on my face because she quickly continued, "It sounds bleak, but it's not. I'm just trying to find the little things that bring joy each day. If Alex is up all night, then he'll take a nap, and Drew and I will bake cookies. What's my alternative? To be bitter or resentful, or take the day that you have?"

Alex's future is still very much uncertain. "I had this pretty picture of preparing Alex for an independent life in a group home, where his brothers could visit, take him home for the weekend—that picture's gone," Lisa said. "I have no idea what's going to happen now—all I know is that he's not going to another hospital or RTF. Our focus in life has completely changed, to knowing he's home and going to be home no matter what."

Lisa believes the problem doesn't lie with these particular facilities, but with the system in general. "For years, I was told Alex would do better in a structured environment with daily psychiatric care and full-time behavior specialists, but he got all that and he decompensated faster than I ever thought possible," she said. She thinks that complicated kids like Alex require a collaborative, multi-disciplinary approach. Instead, she sees clinicians more interested in protecting their turf than working together: behavior specialists who believe all problems can be solved with a behavior plan alone, psychiatrists who shy away from ECT because they haven't used it before. Dr. Wachtel agrees, acknowledging to me during one of Jonah's follow-up visits to KKI that managing dangerous aggression and self-injury in this population is very difficult to do "piecemeal" when "the interdisciplinary team is missing." And sadly, there are very, very few facilities where kids like Alex and Jonah can get medical management by experienced child psychiatrists, ECT if indicated, and appropriate behavioral support. As Lisa laments, "You're at the mercy of whoever you can find to work with."

Still, she's not sorry she tried ECT. In fact, she hopes to try it again in the future, after or in conjunction with the Clozaril Dr. Wachtel suggested. "Balancing Alex's neurochemistry is the only answer," she told me. "Meds don't work, and he can't stabilize himself. ECT is still his only shot." When I pressed her if she would have any regrets if Alex never improved from ECT, she shook her head. "Even if it never works, it did nothing to harm him. He went willingly and happily to Belmont, the staff was respectful and made it as comfortable as possible. He showed no signs of it being aversive. As bad as his behaviors were at that time, we never had to drag him or bribe him. I don't think ECT is something people should be afraid of. It's not scary."

What does scare Lisa is thinking about what will happen to Alex and kids like him once they're grown. "Where are they going to end up?" she asked me, while she picked at her salad. "If I think about it, I get really depressed. We're going to be back in state institutions. These kids are going to be wandering the halls, scratching themselves. I see a very grim and very bleak picture."

CHAPTER 11

Jonah,

August–September 2010

HOW DOES ECT WORK?

AUGUST 31, 2010

"Jonah, stop it!" Marina commands from the last row of our fifteen-person passenger van. "We do not hit!"

My eyes dart to the rearview mirror, trying to assess the situation while driving sixty-five miles per hour up the Atlantic City Expressway. I hear more than I see the ongoing struggle: Jonah yelling, the rustling and muted slaps of Marina's hands blocking Jonah's fists, the dull thump of shoulders and backs bouncing off seats. I scout ahead for a place to pull over that can accommodate our enormous vehicle.

"Ow! Jonah, stop it!"

"I'm pulling over!" I call back, but Marina tells me not to; Jonah has retreated under his blanket.

"Are you okay?" I ask.

"He pulled out a whole handful of Marina's hair," Erika reports from the seat right behind me, like a color commentator narrating a basketball game. Although Jonah's behavior has been great all summer, Erika—like Hilary and the twins—has grown up watching her brother strike the adults in the house and she's used to it. What has always amazed me is that the kids were never afraid of Jonah—even when his tantrums were at their worst, they would just walk around him thrashing on the floor, pause to ask me if they could have a snack or play outside, then continue on their way as if this sort of thing happened in every house. It's true Jonah never hit them, but they did witness many fierce attacks, including one time Jonah grabbed me by the hair and pulled me to my knees, and I couldn't free myself because every time I tried to peel his fingers back he would hit me with his other hand. Finally, I had to ask two-year-old Aaron, in as calm a voice as I could muster, if he could please go find Uncle Matty upstairs and tell him that Mommy needed his help.

"I'm okay," Marina says.

I'm not. After more than four months of almost perfect behavior, of watching Jonah's school disruption graphs flatline at zero, of glowing reports to Dr. Wachtel, of Jonah literally becoming the poster child for ECT, as Dr. Wachtel featured him in psychiatry conferences all over the world—after four months of believing my son would never hurt another person again, the rage is back.

While Jonah had seemed more agitated than usual over the past month, we were all caught off guard by the aggression that resurfaced this week. We were celebrating the last days of summer vacation at our house in Atlantic City, typically one of Jonah's favorite places. But he no longer seemed comfortable in his own skin. Restless, irritable, and demanding, he was unable to enjoy playing in the waves or cruising on our boat. His food obsession was all-consuming and whatever else we offered was immediately rejected. "No roller coaster! No playground! No tube!" Then, two days ago, on the five-mile walk along the boardwalk that either Andy, Marina, or I take with Jonah every morning we're in Atlantic City, Jonah had a pre-ECT caliber meltdown. Marina didn't go into a lot of detail when they returned, shrugging it off as she always did, but he must have attacked her viciously because she ended up accidentally scratching him, leaving an ugly red mark down the side of his right cheek.

Darkness settles through the van as Erika and Hilary, then Jonah, fall asleep. We're going home in the middle of our shore week for two reasons: Jonah has ECT tomorrow morning, and Erika, Hilary, and I are going up to Manhattan with Keri and Declan to celebrate Declan's birthday with a performance of *Wicked* and frozen hot chocolate at Serendipity. Thursday morning we'll drive back to Atlantic City for Labor Day weekend.

But as excited as I've been to take the kids to *Wicked*, right now the New York City trip seems more like an inconvenience I can't get out of. I'd much rather be in the ECT suite tomorrow morning, explaining Jonah's deterioration to Dr. Jaffe myself, instead of sending in my report via Marina. And I'd rather be spending the afternoon with Jonah, watching him carefully to see if this seizure has the therapeutic effect we've witnessed time and time again. I can't imagine enjoying the musical if I can't quiet the persistent question running through my mind: *Has ECT stopped helping Jonah? Is ECT like olanzapine, melatonin, Risperdal—treatments that worked for a few months, then, for whatever reason, simply stopped working?* I keep thinking about "Flowers for Algernon," Charlie's miraculous ascent from mental retardation to genius, and his tragic regression. Now that we've seen how happy Jonah can be, how much he can accomplish, it would be unbearable to watch him backslide to the agitated, unpredictable, violent mess he was before ECT.

SEPTEMBER 4, 2010

Dr. Wachtel, Another bad day—Jonah had an hour-long, off and on fit in which he hit me, Andy, his aide, and his aide's pregnant wife. So sad right now.

I stare at my computer screen for a minute. There's nothing else to say, so I click send.

Although Jonah's treatment didn't have much of an effect this week, Dr. Wachtel doesn't believe ECT has stopped working. She suggested in previous emails that perhaps we tried to stretch out the treatments too soon. At the end of July, we decreased the frequency of Jonah's ECT to once a week from an alternating twice weekly/ once weekly schedule. It seems like such an insignificant change, but Dr. Wachtel warned us many times that some of her other patients regressed significantly after their treatments were reduced— prematurely, as it turned out. Although a couple of patients have been weaned down to one ECT every two weeks, others can't go half that long. One, a nineteen-year-old highly functioning autistic with such severe aggression, self-injury, and suicidality he had been kept in constant restraints at a state hospital before his transfer to KKI, "tried to enucleate himself," Dr. Wachtel wrote, the last time he went longer than five days between treatments.

Enucleate himself? I couldn't begin to imagine what that meant until Dr. Wachtel clarified: he tried to remove his own eye.

Why some patients need more ECT than others is a mystery— twins Gary and David, on the other hand, never needed any maintenance treatments following their acute course of ECT over eight

141

years ago. And this difference isn't limited to the developmentally disabled population. Many adults struggling with depression or bipolar disorder also rely on maintenance treatments at varying intervals to keep their symptoms from returning, like Kitty Dukakis, who gets ECT once a month. Others are able to remain stable on medication. A relative few can even go years without any psychiatric interventions, although the relapse rate for this group is high.

Maintenance therapy of some kind is generally required because the changes that occur in the brain as a result of ECT are, as discussed earlier, transient. Although it's true, as anti-ECT activists constantly complain, that no one can explain exactly how ECT works, the physiological effects of ECT have been well documented. The neuroendocrine theory of ECT focuses on the flood of chemicals released by the brain during the grand mal seizure, including prolactin, thyroid stimulating hormone, adrenocorticotropic hormone and a variety of neuropeptides. These hormones, controlled by the hypothalamus and pituitary, play a role in regulating mood, sexuality, energy, temperature, digestion, and the immune system. Hyperactivity of this hypothalamic-pituitary-adrenal axis—and the excess cortisol released into the bloodstream because of it—is the best-documented neuroendocrine abnormality in serious mood disorders and is often corrected by a course of ECT.[1] The finding that patients who fail to demonstrate an increased prolactin level following ECT (due to variations in charge, electrode placement, or frequency of treatments) show significantly less clinical improvement also supports the hypothesis that such peptides play a role in the mechanism of action of ECT.[2]

Other studies have focused on neurogenesis—the creation of new neurons in the brain—that occurs following the administration of both ECT and antidepressants like Prozac. Contrary to historical conceptions of the adult brain as incapable of growth, research suggests neurogenesis is a lifelong enterprise, at least in healthy individuals. Experts believe that depressed patients stop generating new neurons and that the resumption of neurogenesis may break the depressive episode. ECT and antidepressants release chemicals that promote neuronal cell health and growth, including brain-derived neurotrophic factor (BDNF).[3] Animal studies show that rats given electroconvulsive shock (ECS; the animal equivalent of ECT) exhibit twice as many new neurons as controls.[4] And although there was initially some question as to the functionality of the new neurons, recent research not only found more neurons in rats given ECS, but also found more synapses, indicating the neurons were appropriately connecting with one another.[5] Additional work at Princeton University suggests that these newborn cells play an integral role in the formation of new memories.[6] MRI studies in humans corroborate the animal findings, confirming that post-ECT patients show increased volume in the hippocampus, where most neurogenesis occurs.[7]

Still another theory points to the counterintuitive anticonvulsant properties of ECT, which actually raises the seizure threshold (the amount of electricity needed to stimulate a seizure) over time while shortening seizure length. In fact, ECT has been used to treat status epilepticus, a potentially fatal condition in which the brain won't stop seizing. These anticonvulsant actions include diminished cerebral blood flow and metabolic rate and increased levels of inhibitory neurotransmitters—the combination of which results in an overall drop in neural activity that is correlated to patient improvement.[8]

The oldest hypothesis looks to the same neurotransmitters involved in the mechanism of action of antidepressant medications: dopamine and serotonin, as well as others, including norepinephrine, gamma-aminobutyric acid (GABA), and glutamate. Dopamine's involvement, in particular, is evidenced by the successful use of ECT to treat the rigidity and tremors of Parkinson's disease, symptoms that are caused by a loss of dopamine-generating cells. Promising new work with functional neuroimaging may lead to an understanding of which neurocircuits are abnormal in depression and other neuropsychiatric illnesses. Scientists postulate that ECT may work, in part, by normalizing the activity in specific brain regions or in multiple regions interconnected as "circuits," that are believed to be critical in mood regulation.[9]

These theories aren't mutually exclusive; each may explain part of the body's very complex response to convulsive therapy. Interestingly, no theory of ECT gives any credit to the E, electricity, which has no therapeutic value except as a catalyst for the grand mal seizure in the brain. This seizure is solely responsible for the physiological changes previously described. And, despite the public's intertwined associations of convulsive therapy—Frankensteinian electrodes, singed temples, thrown switches—these seizures can in fact be effectively induced without electricity. When convulsive therapy was first introduced in 1934, doctors injected camphor into their patients to cause seizures. Soon afterward intravenous Metrazol became the preferred agent. By the late 1930s, psychiatrists had begun using electricity because it was cheaper, easier, and faster than the chemical alternatives; the instantaneous action of electricity allayed the fears patients suffered as they waited for the Metrazol to take effect. But scientists are now considering other options, such as magnetic seizure therapy (MST)—in which a high-strength magnetic field is used to induce the seizure—as part of ongoing research into ways of making brain seizures more focal and less generalized, which should reduce side effects while maximizing efficacy.[10]

Right now, I'm less concerned with how Jonah's seizures are induced than how often he should get them. I hate to take anything that seems like a step backward, but if Jonah will do better on the alternating once weekly/twice weekly schedule, then of course that's what he should get. I've idly wondered at times whether we would stick with ECT if it turned out Jonah needed it even more frequently, say three or four times a week. The cost—both in time and money—would be staggering. The mornings of Jonah's treatments, we're out of the house by six thirty, so we can be in front of the locked ECT suite when the doctors and nurses start arriving around seven o'clock. The staff generally lets Jonah go first, even if other patients are waiting when we get there, and the treatment itself is short: an approximately two-minute seizure, followed by about twenty minutes of recovery from the anesthesia. Still, inevitable delays—late staff, the occasional bump by an inpatient—keep us from getting to school much before nine thirty or ten. And although insurance covers the bulk of the expense—$1,200–$1,400 per treatment at our hospital—it doesn't cover all of it. We've paid over $12,000 out of pocket since Jonah's acute course began six months ago.

But we've seen firsthand the costs of managing Jonah's behavior without ECT and those are exponentially greater. Jonah's ten-month stay on the NBU at KKI ran almost $1,000,000—a tab that was, thankfully, picked up by the State of Pennsylvania. Tuition at a residential treatment facility can approach $100,000 a year, and when we were considering an RTF before Jonah started ECT, we assumed that he would have to remain there for the rest of his life. Although we wouldn't be required to shoulder that burden by ourselves, that's still an enormous cost for the school district, the state, and the Federal government to bear.

With respect to time, a few hours a week watching Jonah spin around the ECT suite waiting room or type a list on his iTouch, patiently waiting for Number 1 Doctor so he can get Number 2 Donut, is vastly preferable to the thousands of hours I've spent literally rolling around the floor trying to keep my son from gouging my eyes out, or how many I would pass commuting back and forth to the RTF, stuck at a table, drawing Sesame Street characters while trained aides hovered nearby, waiting to pull Jonah off me when those unpredictable and unmanageable rages overtook him—which, if I can project from past experience, would happen every day. It's clear that even if Jonah became the first person in the world to require daily ECT treatments to keep his mood stable then we would still do it. But that's not even close to what he needs, I remind myself. All we're talking about is going back to three treatments every two weeks.

Before I agree, there's something I need to rule out first. Around the same time that we shifted to weekly ECT, we also added a new medication, memantine, to Jonah's regimen. Dr. Wachtel has found that this glutamatergic agent helps about half her patients extend the time between ECT treatments, and that the other half often respond to a similar medication, riluzole. Abnormally high levels of the neurotransmitter glutamate have been implicated in the speech and socialization impairments of both autism and Alzheimer's disease, for which memantine is most typically prescribed. The role of glutamatergic dysfunction in psychiatric illness in general is an active area of research, and of particular interest to Dr. Wachtel as she seeks adjunctive therapies for patients like Jonah. Although we started with a very low dose that he seemed to tolerate well, perhaps he's having a reaction to the higher level we've built up to over the past month. In any event, even if the memantine isn't hurting Jonah, it's clearly not helping. I ask Dr. Wachtel if we can discontinue it before we change the ECT schedule and she agrees. Since she advises that no tapering is necessary, we stop the memantine immediately.

SEPTEMBER 7, 2010

For years I longed for Jonah to be able to swallow pills. Twice a day, from the time he was in kindergarten, I crushed his pills with a mortar and pestle like a Shakespearian apothecary, carefully coaxed the dust into a dollop of peanut butter, and scraped it on to a piece of bread. Obviously, this wasn't ideal; it was impossible to know how much of the medicine was lost, stuck to the mortar, pestle, dish, knife. And then I'd have to stand over Jonah while he ate the little sandwich, which he was more or less willing to do depending on his mood.

Behavior specialists have developed pill-swallowing protocols for kids with autism, breaking the process down into countless small steps, but I was too intimidated to try to follow one at home. These plans typically start with tiny edibles like sprinkles, Tic Tacs, or even tapioca pearls, and I couldn't even begin to imagine how I would explain to Jonah the difference between chewing and swallowing, especially during those years when he was so easily frustrated. When he went to KKI, I begged his team to run a pill-swallowing protocol with him there, and although they were amenable to it, in the end they didn't have enough time. He came home on the same peanut butter sandwich plan he went in with.

Then, one morning shortly after he was discharged, I gave Jonah one of the chewable children's vitamins I give all my kids. He took it, shoved it to the back of his throat, and swallowed it whole.

When I saw what he was doing, I tried to stop him, afraid he might choke. "Wait, Jonah, chew it—" Then the proverbial lightbulb went on over my head: *You can do that????* I handed him one of his morning pills, pointed down my own throat, and told him to swallow it, which he did. From that day on, he has swallowed all his medicine— sometimes two or three pills or capsules at a time, easily, without even water to wash them down.

I think about that day frequently because it reminds me of something I tend to forget about life with Jonah and even about life in general: sometimes, the hard things turn out to be easy. Once in a while—not often, but occasionally—impediments that seemed insurmountable resolve almost effortlessly.

Like now: amazingly, Jonah's rage is gone. Four days after we stopped the memantine; three days after our Atlantic City vacation ended with an hour-plus fit, the rest of the kids strapped in their seats while Jonah thrashed on the sidewalk, refusing to get in the van; less than a week later, it's as if the regression never happened. Once the memantine cleared his system Jonah's equanimity returned, along with his flexibility, his enthusiasm, and his sense of humor. Despite his longing requests to go back to our shore house, he trooped back to school without protest.

As much of a relief as it is to locate a concrete cause for Jonah's regression, to know that ECT didn't stop working and that we don't need to increase the frequency of his treatments, it's also sobering to consider how quickly his hard-won stability evaporated. ECT quiets Jonah's rage, temporarily releases its capricious grip, but I've come to believe the potential will always be there, waiting for the medication change, the growth spurt, the strep infection that will rouse it once again. It's funny; I look back at the journal I started at the beginning of our ECT journey, my expressed belief that we would someday "beat this thing." But it's only now that we've come so close that I realize we probably never will beat it absolutely and permanently. I only hope that, even if we can't cure Jonah of his rage, we can continue to control it, to plug the inevitable ruptures as quickly as the Little Dutch Boy stopped the leaky dike with his thumb.

Considering these ruptures, I can't help but think of an objection frequently raised by the anti-ECT lobby I find especially peculiar: that ECT creates false euphoria. Psychiatrist Peter Breggin, arguably ECT's most prominent critic, writes, "For a few days or weeks the patient may be euphoric or high as a result of the brain damage [caused by ECT], and this may be experienced as 'feeling better.'"[11]

Never mind that Breggin shamelessly sets up an impossible situation for ECT, defining the terms such that no positive outcome is possible—not only are cognitive impairments, memory loss, headaches, etc., blamed on ECT, but simply "feeling better" is recast as "brain damage." My larger problem with this argument is his assumption that the happiness that returns to most patients following

ECT is unnatural, as opposed to their previous depressed or agitated states, which are somehow more authentic or valuable. No consideration is given to the alternative (and much more intuitive) possibility: that people's natural brain activity can create feelings of false *dysphoria*, of being sad or angry or anxious for no reason. Jonah has attacked me while I was drawing Sesame Street characters for him, while he was watching his favorite videos, while he was walking by the ocean or through his favorite amusement parks. He attacked when no demands were being placed on him and nothing desired was being withheld. Whatever triggered these rages was internal, completely independent of his circumstances or emotional state: there was nothing authentic about them. Far from creating a false euphoria, ECT lifted Jonah's false dysphoria, revealing the happy kid I always knew was underneath.

But setting logic aside for a moment, let's pretend for a moment that Breggin is right and that Jonah's ECT-induced happiness is completely artificial. Does that matter at all?

No, it doesn't. If there's one thing I expect everyone on both sides of this debate can agree on, it's that artificial happiness is vastly preferable to natural rage. For most people struggling with mental illness—the depressed and bipolar adults that comprise the bulk of ECT patients—the choice isn't quite so stark. So it's easier for anti-ECT zealots to muddy the issues with talk of empowerment and authenticity and empathy, to blame anyone and anything they can think of for the debilitating symptoms suffered by patients with mental illness, including the patients' families, society, even the psychiatrists trying to help them. But that's why Jonah, Matthew, Peter, and the other kids I met, as small a group as they are, belong at the crux of the ECT debate. Because once you recognize there are individuals whose negative emotional states are clearly physiological in origin, who simply can't be helped with talk therapy, then how can you draw the line? Who can say that yes, Jonah's unprovoked rage clearly represents a medical condition, but the grandmother who lies unresponsive in the fetal position all day just needs a good psychotherapist?

No one. And Jonah and the grandmother have something else in common: neither would care one iota if their recovered happiness turned out to be as plastic as cheap Mardi Gras beads. It's a meaningless, arrogant, impossible enterprise anyway, teasing apart the tangle of human emotions to knight each one "true" or "false." What matters is the consistency of the emotional state, that stability upon which everything else depends: family, friends, career, independence. Having seen my son drained of joy, bubbling in a constant state of agitation, I can say with absolute certainty that Jonah's entire quality of life will depend on our ability to maintain his happiness, to medically suppress those mysterious, organic rages.

SEPTEMBER 16, 2010

I email Dr. Wachtel with good news this time: Jonah has had virtually no disruptive behaviors of any kind this week. She writes back: "It's so interesting, two of my ECT patients did great on memantine. But no matter, I'm glad Jonah is back to himself."

CHAPTER 12

John

No pseudonyms are used in this chapter.

I'm so grateful to the Dinda family for allowing me to iden-
tify them by name; otherwise, it would be impossible to describe that
gut-wrenching moment in August 2010 when I opened an email from
my tennis partner asking if she could put me in touch with a woman
she had met at a party whose autistic son had such violent behaviors
she was considering a KKI admission. The woman's name was Maude
Dinda.

That name on my computer screen—so familiar, yet utterly unex-
pected—instantly sparked synapses all over my brain: I saw a roller
coaster; a new, pre-fab classroom; an enthusiastic, blond banker
whose amazing leap of faith made me believe anything was possible.

Suddenly, it was 2003 again. Jonah was almost five years old, and
we were trying to decide where he should attend kindergarten. Our
district had several well-respected autism support classrooms, but
Andy and I were captivated by the Magnolia School, a tiny two-class
program that had just opened the previous year. We didn't know
much about the Association Method, Magnolia's intensive language-
based curriculum, but the school had received quite a bit of local and
national buzz, including a spot on *Good Morning America*. We knew
all we felt we needed to know: that Magnolia was started by parents
who had met at an autism conference and decided to act on their
mutual dissatisfaction with the educational options offered to their
developmentally delayed children. Michael Dinda—who had quit his
job in finance to get the school off the ground—was its public face;
when Andy and I went to a fundraiser for Magnolia, he was the one
who took the floor. He told those of us assembled—wealthy work
colleagues, local educators, and parents like us, desperate to get our
kids into his school—a story about his son, John, who was then
about ten years old. Michael and John had gone to an amusement

park and ridden a roller coaster together. Michael recalled the joy on John's face, the fervor with which his barely verbal, barely communicative son signed "more" after each ride, the love that kept Michael on that roller coaster for a dozen turns even though he could barely tolerate it.

I can't remember now why Michael told that story, or how it fit into his larger fundraising message. All I know is that it struck a chord in me. Jonah loved—still loves—roller coasters more than anything in the world, and at five he had just started speaking. Surely this little school specifically designed for a boy who had so much in common with my son was the perfect placement for Jonah. And surely these parents, who had sacrificed so much, researched so exhaustively, set the bar so high, surely they would absolve me of my nearly unbearable guilt. Because not only had I failed to build an educational utopia for my child, but I had often rewound "Big Bird Sings" one more time even though I knew I should be modeling pretend play, forcing Jonah to complete a game of *Hi Ho Cherry-O*, or trying to engage him socially by singing "Old MacDonald" on the swing set.

In the end, we didn't send Jonah to the Magnolia School. The media attention had brought with it a deluge of applications. During the interminable months we waited for the administration to process them all, we met with the autism support coordinators of our public school district who promised to place Jonah with a teacher who was locally famous in her own right for her skill and warmth. After meeting with her and discussing the behavioral supports she would put in place to manage Jonah's aggression, Andy and I decided to withdraw our application from Magnolia. We didn't hear much about it after that, although whenever I passed the YMCA campus that hosted the school I wondered how it was doing, how much bigger it had gotten, if we had made the right choice.

So you can imagine how surprised I was when I finally spoke to Maude Dinda and found out that John's self-injurious and disruptive behaviors had necessitated his removal from the Magnolia School in March of 2004, less than two years after his parents sacrificed everything to open it specifically for him.

"That was the worst period of our lives," Michael told me later. Not only did he feel that Magnolia had failed John, but Michael also felt he had failed the population he had hoped to serve: autistic kids with dangerous behaviors. He believes these children have been virtually outcast by the greater autism community, which would rather embrace inspirational figures like Jason McElwayne, the autistic teen who shot a game-winning basket in 2006. Although Michael had conceived of the Magnolia School as a haven for kids like John, Magnolia's co-founder had a different target population in mind: students with apraxia and other language-related delays. Most of the teachers also supported her agenda—and who could blame them? Every day John came to school, he tore the classroom apart. When the Dindas pulled John out of Magnolia, their involvement with the school also ended.

I was shocked to hear this heartbreaking end to what had seemed in 2003 like an autism fairy tale; devastated to discover the Dindas had spent the next year and a half trying to homeschool John, which in practical terms meant squeezing incidental amounts of instruction around six to eight hours a day of tantrums ("I had a double mattress on the floor so he wouldn't hurt himself," Michael told me. "I would pull the shades. I didn't even get out of my pajamas"). But honestly, I was also a little bit relieved. Because if the Dindas weren't able to stop John's rages after everything they did—and founding Magnolia was only the last and largest in more than a decade of interventions that included diet, vitamins, Secretin, brushing, sensory integration, intensive occupational therapy, and many, many different psychotropic medications—then it was clear that nothing I did or didn't do before ECT would have ended Jonah's aggression. We could have played *Hi Ho Cherry-O* sixteen hours a day, and we still would have ended up in exactly the same place.

A year before she reached out to me, Michael and Maude had placed John in a highly recommended residential treatment facility (RTF)—the same one, in fact, that I had been considering for Jonah. They hoped the greater structure, the behavior experts, and the constant one-on-one attention (which the Dindas, with their two younger children, were unable to provide) would prove therapeutic—but John's behavior worsened. One night, the nurse called them close to midnight to report there was blood in John's urine. When Michael came to take him to the emergency room, he found that John had beaten his own face into a bruised, swollen pulp. He also refused almost all food during his entire admission. Although Maude prepared breakfasts and dinners she knew John would like every day, rather than subject him to the cold, tasteless meals they served at the RTF, by the time he was discharged in October 2010 he was gaunt, his cheeks sunken. He gained thirty pounds within a month of coming home.

Maude still blames herself for those terrible sixteen months. Although John was at his best with support staff that knew him well and could anticipate his sometimes bizarre, and often extreme, reactions, the RTF was specifically designed to prevent the formation of emotional attachments. Each aide had twenty-one kids he or she cycled through, which meant that weeks could go by between repeat assignments. Although this undoubtedly protected the kids from the disruptions of the high turnover rate plaguing this profession, it also left John isolated and friendless.

"Maybe I did know better," Maude told me sadly. "Maybe I just needed a break."

Maude first invited me to her house, only about ten minutes west of ours, two months before John was discharged from the RTF—although it was abundantly clear by that point the placement was a complete failure. The only reason the Dindas didn't pack John up and drive him home immediately was the lack of any viable alternative. They couldn't imagine going back to those months spent on the double mattress in the basement, yet John's behaviors precluded his acceptance at another day school, even one that specifically serviced the autistic population. Michael and Maude wondered, as they had at several points in John's life, whether KKI might be John's best option. We spoke in great detail about Jonah's experience on the NBU: the strategies, the staff, the results. But the discussion switched gears as soon as I told Maude about our success with ECT.

"I remember how cautious you were about bringing it up," Maude laughed recently. Jonah had only been getting ECT for five months at the time of that first conversation, and I hadn't told many of our friends yet, never mind a virtual stranger like Maude. I think I was afraid of encountering in real life the kind of outrage and horror I saw so frequently online and in print during the crash course in ECT

I crafted for myself in the months preceding Jonah's first treatment. Now, of course, Jonah's ECT-induced transformation is one of my favorite topics (right up there with the story of how I ended up with five kids: "I let my husband talk me into going for number four in a moment of weakness"). And even after hundreds of repetitions, not once has Jonah's story ever been met with anything but excitement and compassion. Maybe my friends, neighbors, and casual acquaintances are all accomplished actors, masking their disgust until we part ways, then calling Child Services anonymously with one hand while backing out of my driveway with the other. More likely, the very fact of Jonah shrieking with joy on our boat, pressing his face close to mine with another of his impossible requests ("Mommy. I want one thousand dark red Mike & Ikes. Please."), or helping his father unload our minivan after a typical $500 excursion to Costco— the irrefutable, empirical, documented fact of Jonah now compared to Jonah before—simply eclipses any skepticism or misinformation my listeners may have picked up as engaged members of our *Cuckoo's Nest* culture.

And Maude wasn't just any listener. Like Andy and me, Maude and Michael were exhausted and frustrated after countless failed medication trials. Since the age of five John had been prescribed more than thirty-five different antipsychotics, SSRIs, neuroleptics, and anti-seizure medications, as well as low dose naltrexone, which is typically given to addicts when they detox. Not only did the drugs fail to help, but they often increased John's self-injurious and obsessive-compulsive behaviors. "We just knew pharmacology wasn't the total answer," Maude told me.

Besides, the Dindas were no strangers to intensive medical intervention. Seven months after they pulled John from the Magnolia School, Michael and Maude decided to try plasmapheresis, one of the most cutting edge therapies available at that time. Done under general anesthesia, this procedure involves removing a patient's blood, separating out the plasma in a centrifuge, then replacing it with albumen before infusing the blood back into the patient. Because John had suffered so many strep infections when he was younger, one of his doctors thought his acute obsessive-compulsive behaviors might be the result of Pediatric Autoimmune Neuropsychiatric Disorders

Associated with Streptococcal Infections (PANDAS), in which strep antibodies cross the blood brain barrier and attack the brain. The first of John's two rounds of plasmapheresis, prescribed to remove the strep antibodies, required twice-weekly treatments over the course of eight weeks.

"What's dangerous is not doing something, not acting, because that's what ends tragically," Michael explained to me. And the plasmapheresis did help reduce John's OCD and tics somewhat, enough for him to start at a local private school for autistic students in the fall of 2006. But although John's elaborate rituals had been diffused somewhat—he no longer had to open and close the door dozens of time before leaving the house or lift his fork halfway to his mouth and put it down again so many times that meals could go on for hours—his self-injury was as bad as it had ever been. In 2009, those ceaseless tantrums combined with the resignation of several aides from their home team and John's impending "graduation" from his school (which at that time wasn't licensed to educate kids older than sixteen) to create the surge of despair that swept him into that ill-fitting residential treatment facility.

So the thought of ECT wasn't at all scary to Michael and Maude. "In my mind, ramping John up on Seroquel—that's more scary to me than a physiological intervention that involves some response of his own body," Maude said. "I knew Michael would be all over it."

He was, and with a few emails, I introduced the Dindas to Dr. Kellner and Dr. Wachtel. It took two months to navigate the bureaucratic channels of Mount Sinai and to transition John home from his RTF. On October 11, two days after his discharge, Michael made the first of what would be almost seventy sunrise trips to Manhattan for John's first ECT. John's twenty-year-old cousin came along to help out. Although Michael and Maude were hopeful, they didn't know how John would react. "I assumed this would be a short experiment, because nothing had worked for him before." Maude told me.

But ECT did work, almost immediately. "He went for ECT Wednesday and Friday, and that weekend was amazing," Maude said. "He was smiling, he was relaxed and pleasant—and he hadn't been pleasant for years. And he was talking up a storm—asking Michael to take him to a diner they hadn't gone to in six years, asking to go to church." She paused, trying to convey the magnitude of the change in John's demeanor. Finally, she said, "The furrow between his brows was finally gone."

———

On October 29, 2010, Dr. Wachtel, Dr. Kellner, and other ECT researchers Dr. Max Fink, Dr. Neera Ghaziuddin, and Dr. Dirk Dhossche, presented a symposium on pediatric catatonia at the annual American Academy of Child and Adolescent Psychiatry (AACAP) meeting in New York City. It was a landmark occasion: the first time, after numerous submissions, that AACAP had accepted a panel explicitly endorsing the therapeutic value of ECT. I took the train up from Philadelphia to show my support.

Dr. Kellner was the last one to speak. He followed presentations on the history, misdiagnosis, and treatment of pediatric catatonia. Although the other doctors all spoke at least in part about their experience successfully treating catatonic patients with convulsive therapy, Dr. Kellner's talk was entirely about ECT. He provided an overview for those in the audience who—not uncommon these days—had completed not only medical school, but also psychiatric residency, with little or no education or experience with ECT. One of the slides in his Power Point presentation showed an EEG of a patient mid-seizure with its characteristic pattern of quick, sharp spikes, followed by slow wave activity. I guessed by the date on the EEG, as well as Dr. Kellner's introduction of the slide as belonging to a sixteen-year-old patient, that it was John's. I looked around the room to see if Michael had come in late—Dr. Wachtel had told me that he was planning to attend if he could arrange to have his nephew drive John back to Pennsylvania after his treatment earlier that morning. Sure enough, I saw Michael near the back of the packed audience.

When the presentations were over, I made my way through the crowd to say hello. "That was John's EEG," Michael said excitedly. When I told him that I had assumed as much, he continued: "When I saw that EEG, I couldn't help it—I turned to the woman sitting next to me and said, 'That's my son!'"

I laughed, thinking at first about the perverse world we live in, the parents of kids with severe disabilities—a world in which we take as much pride in a seizure as other parents would take in a touchdown or a piano recital. I had felt the same thrill when Jonah's bloody face appeared on that big screen in the middle of Dr. Wachtel's talk about the use of ECT to treat dangerous behaviors in her patients with developmental disabilities.

Then I decided there was nothing perverse about it. What are parents celebrating when they cheer that score or that sonata but the fulfillment of their children's potential? Those moments when hard work and good fortune coalesce into bright, shiny bubbles of success—well, all kids have them and all parents are overcome by them. Arguably, John's EEG and the transformation it represented were more worthy of public acclaim than any performance by a typical child, simply because there was so much more at stake. After all, this was a boy whose cheekbones had begun to calcify when he was eleven years old to protect his face from his own fists. Now he was back at the day school he had left when an RTF seemed like the only way to keep him safe, and none of the staff could believe he was the same kid.

I couldn't help thinking of Andy's favorite joke: An older gentleman walks into a confessional and says, "Father, I'm a recent widower. Since my wife's death, I've taken up with my twenty-four-year-old secretary. She's a gorgeous blond with enormous breasts. We have sex in exotic positions and in public places. There's no love between us whatsoever, and no hope for marriage." The priest says, "Cease these activities, say three Hail Marys, and all will be forgiven." The man says, "I don't think I'm going to do that." The priest says, "Why not?" The man says, "I'm Jewish." The priest says, "Then why are you telling me this?" And the man says, "I'm telling everybody!" I was so happy for Michael I could have hugged him, right in the middle of that slowly dissipating crowd of psychiatrists still buzzing from Dr. Wachtel's before-and-after pictures. After so much silence, so much grief, why not tell everybody?

———

John's ECT road wasn't without bumps. The lithium typically prescribed along with ECT made him hyper, until Dr. Wachtel lowered his dose, and—like Jonah's experience with memantine— higher doses of the Rilutek that often helps extend the time between treatments left John agitated, so Dr. Wachtel also adjusted that medication. Stretching out his treatments proved especially difficult. The first time the Dindas tried to wean him down to once a week John regressed so badly he had to undergo a second acute course, involving three treatments a week for two weeks. What Maude had assumed would be a "short experiment" stretched out longer than anyone, even Dr. Kellner, anticipated. Whereas Jonah was shifted to maintenance treatments with Dr. Jaffe after only nine sessions, Michael and John were still making that four-hour roundtrip commute to New York City eight months after his first ECT.

"I would drive to New York once a week forever if the benefits would stick," Michael told me. But it turned out he didn't have to. By August 2011, John had very slowly been weaned again to weekly treatments and the Dindas transitioned to Dr. Jaffe.

This is where John's story overlaps with Jonah's, with Matthew's, with Paul's, Gary's, David's, Sam's—in his parents hopes for the future, now that his self-injurious and destructive behaviors are almost completely gone. Given their tremendous initiative when it came to the Magnolia School, it didn't surprise me at all to hear that the Dindas wanted more for John than another RTF "holding tank," or a sheltered workshop that's nothing more than "a warehouse with tables and chairs." They believed they could use the money the state spent to support John to design a better option: maybe a staffed home with other autistic peers, one that would challenge its residents and involve them in the community, through jobs, volunteer work, and frequent outings.

I believed them, too. And I couldn't imagine a happier ending for Jonah's story than a loving group home established by the Dindas. But first Michael and Maude needed to get over the post-traumatic-stress-disorder-like reactions that caused their hearts to race every time one of their kids clapped or they heard some other sudden, loud noise that in the past indicated a tantrum was coming. "I can't get over the feeling that this just can't stay," Maude told me. "I think my psyche is trying to brace itself for a regression."

But maybe her psyche was relaxing just a little. Although Maude still wouldn't take John by herself to his beloved movies every Saturday and Sunday, she did take him for long walks on the nature trail near their house. "I need to live with him longer this way first," she explained. She and Michael were both amazed at how each happy day cracked John's world just that much wider. So, appropriately enough, John's story ends for now right where it began for me—with roller coasters. As much as John has always loved them, he hadn't been to an amusement park in years because of his unmanageable rages. But in June 2011, his school organized a trip to Dorney Park. Michael and Maude were so concerned about how the overstimulation, lack of structure, and change of routine might challenge John's newfound stability that they asked one of his home aides to drive up after lunch in case John needed to leave the park early. But before the aide could leave, John's teacher called Maude. "Don't come," she said. "John is having a great time."

CHAPTER 13

The ECT Controversy

OCTOBER 5, 2010

It's amazing how fast we re-normalize. For more than eight years we were used to our son attacking us, sometimes several times a day; now, seven months after we started ECT, we're used to the opposite. When, as happens occasionally—maybe a couple of times a month—Jonah takes a half-hearted smack at one of us, it's surprising: *Oh right*, we think, *you used to do that*.

Not that our struggles are by any means over. Jonah turns twelve in three months, and as we stare down puberty's barrel, we wonder what explosions lie in wait for us when it goes off. I think sometimes about Dr. Kolevzon's disclosure that most of his aggressive patients were unable to live at home once they became teenagers, and I say a brief prayer that ECT will help us through what may be the most difficult years of Jonah's life, but I don't dwell on it much. Like the other parents in this book, I am just happy to celebrate the peace that has been restored to my home (or, I should say, *relative* peace; with eight kids in the house, who am I kidding?). I celebrate the freedom to take my son to the store, to the barber, to the zoo without help. And I celebrate above all else Jonah's happiness, now that he is largely free of the irrational, unpredictable, uncontrollable rages that would regularly crash through his mind like some kind of cerebral tsunami.

Given the impressive improvements in Jonah, Matthew, Paul, Gary, David, Sam, John, and more young people than I had room to include here, it surprises, saddens, and yes, scares me to hear the anti-ECT movement call for ECT to be banned. I want to believe that most of these cries come from people who have no idea how much ECT has helped us reclaim our children, but honestly, I don't think that would matter to those groups' most strident followers. Linda Andre opens the last chapter of her book *Doctors of Deception: What They Don't Want You To Know About Shock Treatment* with a quote from a letter to the FDA written by Ed van Hoom: "The argument that electroshock sometimes helps people is in our view a non-valid argument. We live in a civilized society in which not all the things that help people are allowed."

I find this to be a bewildering position. There are plenty of people who believe they were harmed by any number of things, yet don't demand those things be denied to others who may be helped by them. Taking another example from the world of autism, consider the parents who believe their children's autism was caused by a reaction to vaccines. Not once have I ever heard one of these parents argue for vaccines to be banned for everyone; rather, they argue for the right not to vaccinate their own kids. Still, their claims provoked a mighty response from the medical establishment, as the AMA, the CDC, the NIH and other organizations released study after study rejecting any link between autism and immunizations.

So why haven't the NIH or the National Institute of Mental Health (NIMH) marshaled any of their considerable resources against the inflamed rhetoric of the anti-ECT groups? I know that the status of ECT in our society doesn't present the threat to public health posed by unvaccinated children, but neither should we diminish the impact it has had, and continues to have, in the mental health arena. Every year, 100,000 patients receive ECT—a population comprised almost exclusively of depressed and bipolar adults. But given the success stories reported in these pages, supported by research coming out of such leading institutions as KKI and the University of Michigan, it seems likely that number will grow—that it *should* grow. Right now, the number of autistic individuals in this country is 730,000 and rising, as diagnostic rates have soared to the point that a staggering one out of every one hundred fifty kids is diagnosed with a spectrum disorder—and up to a third of those, according to recent research, will exhibit aggressive and/or self-injurious behavior. How bad are these behaviors? Severity varies across individuals, but a 2005 British study found that over 16 percent of all the developmentally delayed young people in the London borough of Camberwell had a "marked problem," as opposed to a "minor problem," with aggression. If this percentage is representative of the autistic population as a whole, it translates into a population of violent autistics potentially 370,000 strong: larger than all but eleven of the standing armies in the entire world.[1] And that doesn't even include the 11.5 percent of the individuals in the study whose self-injury was a "marked problem." I'm leaving this latter group out of my calculations simply because it's not indicated in the study how many, if any, subjects were counted in both categories.[2]

The financial implications are mind-boggling. Aging parents can hardly be expected to manage such behaviors in children as big or bigger than they are. And the mental health system is completely unprepared to step in. Even if only half this population is dangerous enough to themselves or to others to require inpatient care—a conservative estimate, as it doesn't take that high a level of aggression in an adult male to necessitate his removal from the community—providing that structured, supported physical environment isn't cheap. In 2010 the Federal government reimbursement rate for inpatient psychiatric care was $615 a day, which calculates to almost $225,000 per patient, or over forty billion dollars a year. And that's just the base rate. It doesn't include the one-on-one aides, crisis teams, or other supports required to manage especially violent behavior. If only 50,000 of that 370,000 are so extremely aggressive and/or self-injurious they require around-the-clock, one-on-one supervision, that still necessitates the hiring of over 200,000 additional aides—a figure equivalent to a quarter of the nation's entire police force.

Of course, staffing needs could be reduced, but only if we resort to much less humane tactics, such as heavy sedation or physical restraint, as many facilities do now to manage their most intractable patients. In 2006, the Office of Inspector General for the Department of Health and Human Services released a report that confirmed that 104 psychiatric patients died between 1999 and 2004 while being restrained—and acknowledged that, because of drastic underreporting, the actual number could be much higher. Eight years earlier, the *Hartford Courant* published an investigative series on restraint deaths in psychiatric facilities, reporting that the majority of the victims were children and teenagers. Incidentally, nothing in these statistics reveals whether or not restraint was actually indicated. As a parent who has had to restrain her son; who has watched him restrained by teachers, aides and therapists, I can attest that—as much as we want to believe this is a sadistic strategy used by overworked and undertrained employees—sometimes safety demands it. When a child has already detached his own retinas, or broken a teacher's nose, it is irresponsible to risk further injury by allowing his rages to go unchecked. Restraint is all that's left once you follow the lead of the anti-ECT organizations and reject the stabilizing potential of ECT and psychotropic medications.

If ECT's tremendous impact alone weren't sufficient to provoke a more decisive defense from our nation's largest medical organizations, you might think they would feel compelled to correct the bad science continually promulgated by anti-ECT groups. Philosophically, the movement is based on a theory that has been conclusively rejected by the mainstream medical establishment: that mental illness is not a disease with a biological origin, like diabetes, that needs to be treated medically, but purely a result of environmental factors. In other words, people are depressed because they're in debt or their marriages are failing or they're unemployed. And all these depressed people need are sympathetic ears and good psychotherapists.

This argument was most comprehensively articulated by Thomas Szasz in his 1960 book, *The Myth of Mental Illness*. Szasz categorically rejects "biological considerations as explanations" for mental illness, writing, "We now deny moral, personal, political, and social controversies by pretending that they are psychiatric problems: in short, by playing the medical game."[3] His interpretation of psychiatric symptoms as cries for help by the oppressed against the oppressors resonated fiercely during a decade in which social hierarchies were challenged and in some cases, toppled ("Fix the power," as Jonah might say). And his beliefs are still appealing to many people in their emphases on personal responsibility and empowerment. After all, if someone you loved struggled with incapacitating mental illness, how nice would it be to believe that all he really needed was to learn "to enlarge his choices by enhancing his knowledge of himself, others, and the world about him, and his skills in dealing with persons and things"?[4] No meds with their catalogue of side effects, no ECT, no hospitals, no "interventions which curtail the client's autonomy."

Not every anti-ECT activist necessarily subscribes to this anti-biological view personally, but that argument is raised again and again by the most public voices. The largest organized anti-ECT group, for example, is the Church of Scientology. Scientologists' rejection of the entire psychiatric profession is hardly news—is it possible that anyone in this country missed the heated clash between Brooke Shields and Tom Cruise in 2005 over Shields' use of Paxil to treat her post-partum depression?—but to let the Church speak for itself, I took this from the official website: "There is categorically no evidence that diseases such drugs [antidepressants, stimulants, etc.] claim to treat even exist—which is to say, it's all an elaborate and deadly hoax."

And the Scientologists aren't alone. Leonard Roy Frank, the ECT "survivor" who gets my vote for the most creative, visceral, even poetic condemnations of ECT (calling it, among many, many, *many* other things, "a crime against the spirit and a desecration of the soul") claimed at a 2001 public hearing on ECT before the Mental Health Committee of the New York State Assembly, "There's still nothing in the way of scientific evidence to support the brain-disease notion."[5]

You might think the American public could be trusted to question the credibility of extremists like Frank and the Scientologists. But what happens when the same arguments are repeated by a Harvard-educated psychiatrist who has authored sixteen books and been called to testify in countless trials supporting plaintiffs who claimed they were injured by psychotropic drugs or ECT?

Dr. Peter Breggin has made a career out of attacking medical treatments for mental illness, such as drugs and ECT. Like many of his fellow anti-ECT activists, he also insists, "there is no evidence that any of the common psychological or psychiatric disorders have a genetic or biological component." Amazingly enough for anyone who has ever spent thirty seconds with a child on the spectrum, he includes autism in this category: "It's hard for me to grasp how a biochemical defect could specifically drive a child to withdraw from other people and to treat them wholly without love or affinity, while sometimes maintaining a normal intelligence or even special intellectual gifts. On the other hand, it's very easy for me to see how an inherently intelligent child, treated as an object, would learn to treat others in the same fashion."[6] I almost fell over when I read that passage. Although the "refrigerator mom" theory, popularized in the 1950s, was one of the first attempts to posit an etiology of autism, psychologist Bernard Rimland emphatically denounced it back in 1964. Until I read Breggin's rehash, the only contemporary references I'd seen to this hypothesis described it as exactly what it is: a heartbreaking, misguided, dangerous anachronism that served for many years to justify removing autistic children from their parents' care. Breggin, incidentally, added an interesting twist to this theory, blaming any neurological impairments suffered by autistic children on the drugs pushed by their parents. In so doing he revealed a shocking blindness to what is, in all likelihood, the true causative relationship: that parents resort to drugs to control dangerous and debilitating behaviors caused by neurological impairments.

After reading the same argument echoed by Frank, Breggin, and the Scientologists, I was forced to wonder whether there might be a shred of truth in it. Was it possible that even a small group of respected doctors and researchers believed autism, schizophrenia, and the major mood disorders were caused solely by environmental factors? Could this be interpreted as a true division in the medical community, no matter how unbalanced the sides might be?

But there is no division. Neuroscientist David Eagleman dismisses the idea that these illnesses are purely psychic constructs, not caused by underlying brain dysfunction, as one that "nowadays makes little sense."[7] Although it's true that no mental illness has the simple genetic mechanism of diseases such as cystic fibrosis, which is caused by a mutation in one particular gene, it's now commonly acknowledged that mental illness—just like diabetes and cancer—requires both a genetic predisposition and an environmental trigger. In addition to family and adoption studies, the genetic component has been consistently established by that gold standard of genetic research, the twin study, in which the rates of conditions under investigation in identical twins (who share 100 percent of their DNA) are compared to those in fraternal twins (who only share 50 percent). This type of study successfully parses out genetic from environmental influences, since both types of twins face very similar environmental influences if raised in the same family. And twin studies have shown a significant genetic component in autism, depression, bipolar disorder, and schizophrenia.[8]

Now the question in research labs around the world has shifted from *whether* these disorders have a genetic basis to *which* particular genes are involved—and researchers agree that most mental illnesses are polygenic, the product of several genes, called "susceptibility genes." These genes have a cumulative effect: the more variants an individual has, the more likely he or she is to develop the

disease. Scientists have traced both autism and catatonia to mutations on chromosome 15, which is also involved in the regulation of
gamma aminobutyric acid (GABA) an important neurotransmitter
in the brain.[9] Potential culprits also lie on other chromosomes, including 7, 16, and X—which would help explain why four out of five
autistics are males.[10] Bipolar research points to susceptibility points
on chromosomes 18, 4, and 21, and major depression likely involves
mutations on chromosome 12.[11] Schizophrenia may involve ten or
more genes, including a variant on chromosome 15, which, as mentioned above, is of particular interest to researchers studying autism
and catatonia.[12] In fact, the same individual gene mutation may be
involved in the expression of completely different illnesses, depending on the other genes involved.

———

Last week I saw an episode of the TV show *Private Practice*
that left me sobbing on my treadmill. It featured an aggressive, self-
injurious autistic boy and his single mother. Various medical and behavioral protocols supervised by one of the doctors in the practice
had failed to help, so his mother gave him medical marijuana that
had been prescribed for her migraines by a different doctor in the
same practice. Although the marijuana did noticeably help the boy,
and the doctors were familiar with recent studies suggesting that
marijuana may be effective in treating these symptoms, the doctors
were appalled that the mother had given it to her son, and demanded
she stop immediately. Later, the boy ended up in the emergency
room, after ingesting pot laced with PCP that his mother had bought
on the street in her attempt to duplicate the effect of the medical
marijuana.

Being a big fan of *Private Practice* and its sister show, *Grey's
Anatomy*, I really thought I knew what would happen next: the
doctors would realize that although medical marijuana was an un-
orthodox treatment for autism, what really mattered—and was un-
disputed in the episode—was that the boy's quality of life, as well
as his mother's, was drastically improved by it. And although it was
completely natural for the doctors to be concerned about the impact
of pot on the developing brain, the side-effect profile for marijuana is
actually pretty benign when compared to the hard-core antipsychotics that hadn't worked for this patient anyway. The doctors would

be reminded of the importance of thinking outside the box, the boy would be stabilized, the mom's stress migraines would disappear. Everyone wins.

But no. What actually happened, what I still can't believe happened, was that the doctors called the cops, the mom was arrested, and the kid was shipped off to social services. The end.

What's remarkable about this show was that no viable alternatives were presented to the family. Although they were quick to reject the marijuana that had so helped the boy, the doctors were unable to come up with even one potential replacement to ease his symptoms. In this way, the episode reminded me of anti-ECT groups who denounce ECT, but have nothing else to recommend for my son if, God forbid, their lobby succeeds in banning it.

Let me say one thing here that perhaps I should have said on the very first page, but thought it was so obvious it didn't need to be made explicit: no parents *want* to shock their kids. We don't want to repeatedly put our kids under general anesthesia, inject them with muscle relaxants, or introduce anything to the brain that wasn't there to start with. Neither do we want to give them psychotropic medication, to constantly adjust their brain chemistries in desperate attempts to stop their dangerous behaviors while at the same time making them fat, thirsty, tired, agitated, restless, and who knows what other bizarre and distressing and possibly permanent side effects they often can't tell us about.

Similarly, the doctors who perform ECT aren't Frankensteins who would attach electrodes to the forehead of every wayward child in America if it weren't for the ceaseless vigilance of groups like ect. org. Dr. Kellner said it best in a Grand Rounds he gave at KKI that I attended last May. He told the assembled group of psychiatrists, medical students, nurses, and other mental health care professionals that he wasn't, as they might assume, an ECT zealot. Rather, he considers himself an ECT *advocate* who believes ECT should be available to those patients who need it (he confided in me afterwards that he is, in fact, a zealot about something else: barefoot running). And this description applies to every psychiatrist I met during this project: Dr. Wachtel, Dr. Ghaziuddin, Dr. Jaffe. I never considered, even for a moment, that these doctors were motivated by anything but the best interests of their patients.

The problem is, there's no warm and fuzzy treatment for our kids. It's not like our choice is between ECT and hug therapy. As a group, I believe the parents in this book may have tried every single alternative therapy ever bandied about the autism community like beach balls at a rock concert: diets, vitamins, fatty acids, antivirals, antifungals, chelation, auditory integration training, hyperbaric oxygen therapy, brushing—with absolutely no success. Our only other option, if ECT ever becomes unavailable, is to try again with psychotropic medication, which many anti-ECT activists consider just as abusive (Peter Breggin refers to the effect of such drugs as "chemical lobotomy"). So I ask: *What would they have us do?*

I guess I'm not the first person to ask this question because Breggin addresses it directly:

> When I criticize toxic psychiatry, people often ask urgently about my alternatives. They want to know what I have to offer that's better. . . . But the request for specific alternatives expresses the narrowness of our vision. . . . Once we have begun to think in such a manner, we are already on the wrong track. We are turning for a solution to the critic, and that is bound to increase our feelings of helplessness, fear, and dependence. We are seeking *the answer*, which is likely to be too simple, too shallow, and in all likelihood too authoritarian and self-limiting. We overlook the truth that rejecting bad theories and practices is, in and of itself, a sufficient blessing—one that liberates us to imagine and to implement better ways of healing.[13]

Helplessness? Helplessness is watching your own child put his head through a window, smash the furniture, or stand frozen like a statue for days. It's trying to keep calm while you pry his fingers out of your hair or off your arm while trying not to get bitten, kicked, or punched. It's knowing there is absolutely nothing you can do to end the spells but wait for them to pass.

I think it's telling that the two most vocal ECT "survivors" lobbying today both claim they never needed ECT in the first place because they weren't really sick. Linda Andre writes, "I've been told that I worried out loud to a friend that I might undermine my successful career because I'd internalized my mother's messages about how worthless I was."[14] A visit to a psychiatrist and the machinations of a traitorous brother led to Andre's hospitalization in the early 1980s, where she was threatened with commitment if she didn't consent to ECT.

Leonard Roy Frank's account is even more harrowing. In 1962 his parents committed him to a San Francisco psychiatric hospital for nothing worse than growing a long, bushy beard; adopting a hippie, vegetarian lifestyle; and rejecting his conservative upbringing in favor of the spiritual principles of Gandhi. There he was given fifty insulin coma treatments and thirty-five sessions of ECT, the combination of which he called "the most devastating, painful and humiliating experience of my life."[15]

I have tremendous sympathy for these stories. There's no doubt that the history of psychiatry, like so many other professions, is littered with abuse. Some was no doubt due to malicious doctors, but most arose from the traditional dearth of effective treatments for debilitating mental illness that drove psychiatrists to try all kinds of bizarre—and, arguably, inhumane—treatments, including spinning, blistering, and almost drowning patients. If Andre and Frank want to pass a law prohibiting people from being forcibly subjected to invasive medical procedures *they don't need*, I'll gladly vote for it. I'd be very surprised if such a law weren't already in place.

But that's not the law they want to pass. These activists, who admit they know nothing about what it's like to suffer from incapacitating mental illness, want to ban the therapy that has helped millions of people around the world enjoy happy, productive lives. It's the one therapy that stopped Matthew from punching himself in the face; that snapped Paul's catatonia; that stopped Jonah's violence.

And anti-ECT groups are controlling the dialogue in this country—despite their shaky science, despite scare tactics that at times unapologetically misrepresent the treatment and those who have had it. Consider the movement's adoption of Sylvia Plath as a posthumous spokesperson, as described in a 2001 article in the *Sunday Times of London* (proudly re-posted on the ect.org website) by Kathy Brewis:

> The horror stories surrounding electroconvulsive therapy (ECT) abound. This is the poet Sylvia Plath's grimly eloquent account

from her autobiographical novel *The Bell Jar*: "Don't worry," the nurse grinned down at me. "Their first time, everybody's scared to death." I tried to smile, but my skin had gone stiff, like parchment. Doctor Gordon was fitting two metal plates on either side of my head. He buckled them into place with a strap that dented my forehead, and gave me a wire to bite. I shut my eyes. There was a brief silence, like an indrawn breath. Then something bent down and took hold of me and shook me like the end of the world. Whee-ee-ee-ee, it shrilled, through an air crackling with blue light, and with each flash a great jolt drubbed me till I thought my bones would break and the sap fly out of me like a split plant. I wondered what terrible thing it was that I had done.

Yes, that is the way the Plath character, Esther Greenwood, describes her first experience with unmodified ECT, which was administered without anesthesia. But I can only assume that Brewis stopped reading at that point or she would know that, later in the book, Dr. Nolan tells Esther, "That was a mistake. It's not supposed to be like that. If it's done properly, it's like going to sleep." And if she read through to the end, Brewis might have felt obliged to report that after a failed suicide attempt and a long hospitalization that included talk therapy and insulin treatments, it was actually ECT that broke Esther's debilitating depression. After waking up from the first of a series of treatments prescribed by Dr. Nolan, Esther observes, "All the heat and fear had purged itself. I felt surprisingly at peace. The bell jar hung, suspended, a few feet above my head. I was open to the circulating air."

Despite these persistent inaccuracies, anti-ECT propaganda has succeeded in making the treatment increasingly difficult to obtain. As I've mentioned, five states prohibit the administration of ECT to minors. Other states, such as New Jersey, Montana, and New York, have passed restrictions requiring patients to consult with additional doctors and, in some cases, lawyers. Pending regulatory action by the FDA could further reduce, or even eliminate, access to ECT. ECT machines have been considered Class III medical devices, the riskiest group, since 1979, when complaints from former patients caused the FDA to list memory loss and cognitive impairment as possible side effects. The APA has been trying to reclassify the machines as Class

II ever since, and although the FDA agreed to this in 1982, the classification never was changed. The machines have remained in a kind of federal limbo—still in Class III, but not required, because of their grandfathered status (ECT predates by several decades the FDA's regulation of medical devices, which began in 1976), to go through the Pre-Market Approval (PMA) application required of devices in this category. This process involves the submission of extensive proof of safety studies, often including clinical trials performed by the manufacturers.

Now with deadlines looming, the FDA must decide whether to reclassify ECT devices or force the manufacturers to document the safety of their machines. The owners of these companies, none of whom are psychiatrists, have already stated that they have neither the money nor the expertise to provide these trials. Although the APA's 2001 Task Force Report on Electroconvulsive Therapy cites hundreds of studies in support of the safety and efficacy of ECT, the FDA requires that PMAs be filed by the manufacturers themselves. Although I can't imagine the FDA pulling all ECT devices off the market, that's exactly what's supposed to happen if the manufacturers can't supply the necessary data.

Linda Andre, who has been very involved in this process, points out in her book how the overwhelming majority of letters submitted to the FDA from former ECT patients have been opposed to reclassification. She writes about a 1982 hearing where ten ECT "survivors" got up to testify to FDA officials that they suffered amnesia from their treatments, yet not one satisfied patient was there to represent the other side. She suggests that such patients don't really exist.

But considering all the Holocaust imagery pushed by the anti-ECT camp, it's hardly surprising that professional adults aren't lining up to admit their episodes of mental illness were resolved through ECT. And the families I know who have chosen silence over testimony haven't done so because ECT failed their children—quite the opposite. One parent didn't want her child's story featured in this book because the Church of Scientology had already tried to have her son removed from her custody for giving him the ECT that saved his life when he developed malignant catatonia. Another parent, whose son spent his days strapped to a bed in an institution before ECT, was afraid that any publicity might jeopardize his maintenance treatments in their conservative state. I feel for these families because I understand their fear as much as I share their hope, their joy, and their tremendous relief that after all the doctors, and all the protocols, and all the failures, something finally worked.

Still, several former ECT patients have spoken up, especially in the past ten years, about their experiences and challenged the public to reconsider their views of this stigmatized procedure. I've mentioned a few of them earlier: surgeon and National Book Award winner Sherwin Nuland, psychologist Martha Manning, writer and mental health advocate Andy Behrman, and former Massachusetts First Lady Kitty Dukakis have all written books wholly or in part about how ECT resolved the mental illnesses that left them, in some cases, completely incapacitated. Dukakis still gets maintenance treatments to stave off her depression, eight years later.

And now, new names to add: Jonah, Matthew, Paul, Gary, David, Sam, John. Obviously not the celebrities typically preferred as spokespeople, like other ECT luminaries Carrie Fisher, Tammy Wynette and Dick Cavett, who stated in 1992, "In my case ECT was miraculous. My wife was dubious, but when she came into my room afterward, I sat up and said, 'Look who's back among the living.' It was like a magic wand." If anything, these kids are anti-celebrities, whose dangerous and unpredictable behaviors kept them—until recently—cloistered from public view. Maybe I shouldn't be surprised that Peter Breggin and the other anti-ECT activists quoted here seem oblivious to the dark, mysterious misfirings in some brains that occur no matter how much love, patience, and understanding are showered upon them; misfirings like those that caused twenty-one-year-old autistic Adam Wilson to stab his father to death in August 2010, or that caused twenty-eight-year-old Jeff Apple, also autistic, to smash his head against a tile floor hard enough to kill himself in 1990 (as recounted in Patricia Apple's memoir, *Spinning Straw: The Jeff Apple Story*). After all, I'm sure a lot of what some of my closest friends and family members read in this book may be news, even to them. We, the parents of these children, want to protect them from the startled, curious, judgmental eyes of the world. We don't talk about them; we don't take them out; and the only time anyone hears anything about them is when tragedy strikes.

Or now, when it's so dramatically, so decisively averted. You're more likely to find us out than in these days. If you're ever in Costco or BJ's, look for us. Jonah likes to spin in the refrigerated section. Due to his altered vestibular system, he can spin like Scott Hamilton on skates if we let him kick his shoes off—which we know we shouldn't, but we let him do sometimes, since he asks so nicely: "Daddy, I want shoes off. Please." You may be alarmed at how fast he moves, balanced on the ball of one foot, but don't worry—he never falls.

Epilogue, January 26, 2011
THE FDA HEARING

Thank you, members of the panel. My name is Amy Lutz. My son Jonah suffers from autism and rapid-cycling bipolar disorder. Until last March, he was plagued by frequent, unpredictable and violent rages, during which he would pound himself in the face, like this . . . until he looked like this. . . .

I paused to hold up the bloody pictures of Jonah I had taken following his discharge from KKI, when the state insurance company had failed to deliver even half the hours of home support its own experts had determined Jonah would need to maintain the gains he had made on the NBU—only these prints of the photos were three feet long and two feet high. I wanted to make sure that every member of the Neurological Devices Panel of the Medical Devices Advisory Committee of the FDA got a good look at those disturbing images.

I'm showing you these pictures because I need you to understand the state of crisis we lived in for the better part of a decade. Because even worse than what he would do to himself was what Jonah would do to others when he was in one of these states. He broke a teacher's nose when he was six years old, and by the time he was ten—when these pictures were taken—his almost daily attacks left me, his teachers, and his aides bruised, scratched, and bitten.

Behind the lectern, I could feel my knees trembling. Somewhere deep inside, the debate champion I had been once upon a time mocked my nervousness. When I was in college, I had gotten up almost every weekend to argue, often about topics I knew nothing about, sometimes in front of hundreds of spectators. But there was so much more at stake this time than whether I would take home another silver plate—this panel would advise the FDA whether ECT machines should be reclassified as Class II medical devices.

We tried everything to control Jonah's aggression, including every alternative treatment ever promoted by the autism community: a gluten- and casein-free diet, vitamin cocktails, B12 injections, auditory integration training, hyperbaric oxygen therapy. When none of these helped, we tried pharmacological interventions: antipsychotics, antidepressants, beta-blockers, anticonvulsants, lithium, stimulants. During an almost year-long hospitalization at the Kennedy Krieger Institute, Jonah was briefly stabilized on a combination of lithium and Abilify. But only a few weeks after he came home, the behaviors returned, and less than a year after discharge they were worse than ever.

These fits came upon him under any and all circumstances—while he was doing schoolwork, eating meals, even watching his favorite videos. In October of 2009, Jonah threw a tantrum in the car, lashing out at his eighty-year-old grandfather, who was driving. While trying to restrain Jonah in the confines of our minivan, my husband accidentally broke Jonah's arm. We were faced with the crushing realization that it was no longer safe to keep Jonah at home—not for him, and not for his four younger siblings. At ten, Jonah was already over one hundred pounds, and puberty loomed around the corner—a time when the violent behavior of autistic boys typically grows much worse. I didn't want to imagine what 'much worse' would look like for Jonah, but I couldn't stop thinking about Kent State professor Trudy Steuernagel, who was beaten to death in 2009 by her nineteen-year-old autistic son.

It hadn't been easy to get a spot to testify. Despite my intense interest in ECT, I only found out about the meeting less than two weeks before, when a friend sent me the link to an article in *The Wall Street Journal* that vaguely referred to an upcoming FDA hearing. A search on the FDA website turned up the public docket—along with the deadline to apply to speak at the meeting, which had passed a few days earlier. I called and emailed the contact person, trying my best to sound calm and rational as I explained on his voicemail how imperative it was that the panel hear about Jonah and the other kids I'd met whose quality of life depended solely on their access to ECT. I was sympathetic to this poor public servant, besieged—or so I imagined—by hysterical callers, such as those who left comments in the electronic docket calling ECT "draconian," "cruel," and "unethical," similar to "forced drilling of holes in people's heads," when what mental health patients really needed were "true treatments . . . such as meditation and yoga." But my sympathy evaporated as he failed to return even one of my messages.

Frustrated, I turned to the best strategy I had for getting people's attention: I sent my bloody pictures of Jonah to my senators, my representative, the Commissioner of Food and Drugs, even to a state representative who almost certainly had little involvement with the FDA but who was a consistent champion of the autistic community. I discovered soon after posting them, however, that because of the anthrax scare Congressional mail now undergoes such thorough screening that it can take up to two weeks to reach the intended recipient. None of the senators or representatives I was hoping would help get me in front of that panel would even receive my pictures (or my letter, or the study I included showing no long-term cognitive impairment in adolescents given ECT) until it was too late.

Being Jewish, I'm not a huge believer in the New Testament. However, there's a lesson from the Book of Matthew whose relevance and insightfulness has frequently surprised me: *Ask and ye shall receive.* I was so preoccupied with my quest that I could speak of little else—and my friends, it turned out, had great suggestions. One told me to research what Congressional committee has oversight of the FDA, then call and ask to speak with a staffer who works on regulatory issues. It didn't take me long to reach the Health, Education, Labor and Pensions (HELP) Committee or to discover that Pennsylvania's own Senator Robert Casey serves on that committee. Soon, I had two congressional aides pressuring the FDA to, at the very least, call me back.

Another friend introduced me to a lobbyist friend of his, who suggested I reach out to any big organizations that supported ECT. I had told him about my failed attempts to contact CNN (yes, I'll admit it: I emailed Sanjay Gupta), the *New York Times*, the *Washington Post*, and the *Huffington Post*, and how stunned I still was at the profound lack of media interest in a story that had all the buzzwords reporters seemingly dream about these days: *autism, Scientology, kids, cures.* He said that when reporters want to attach a face to a story, they typically contact organizations, because you never know if a random person who calls or emails a newspaper is insane or not.

"The APA supports the reclassification of ECT," I mused out loud.

"Call their media department," he advised. "Just tell them Jonah's story. Let them know that you're available for press interviews."

This turned out to be the most helpful suggestion of all. The APA was not only very interested in Jonah's story, but the organization was sponsoring several witnesses at the FDA meeting, one of whom had just canceled. I found out two days before the meeting that I could take her spot.

But we didn't need to place Jonah in a residential facility after all. In March of 2010, we decided to try ECT, because we knew it had been used successfully at Kennedy Krieger on kids with dangerous behaviors who didn't respond to medication. Less than a month later, Jonah's aggression was almost completely gone. Gone. And ECT stopped his rages without any of the personality changes or cognitive impairments you've heard a lot about during this hearing. Quite the opposite. According to Jonah's school data, before ECT, he acquired an average of seven new skills per month. In December 2010, he acquired fifty-two new skills.

It was a crazy forty-eight hours: not only did I have to write my testimony and rush production of two-foot by three-foot posters of those bloody pictures of Jonah, but I had to pack my entire family for our first trip together on a plane in over four-and-a-half years. The very night of the FDA meeting, we were all scheduled to fly to Orlando for five days in Disney World. We had finally planned that escape to sunny skies I had dreamed about every winter. But, since the FDA hadn't released a schedule for the two-day meeting, I had no idea whether I'd be able to make it back in time for our seven p.m. flight.

It didn't matter. Andy and I both agreed that testifying was more important than Disney World. If necessary, Andy and Marina would take the five kids down to Orlando without me, and I would follow them on a later flight. The irony wasn't lost on any of us. At the very moment my family would be walking through the gates of the Magic Kingdom, on a trip that was unquestionably possible because of ECT and ECT alone, the FDA panel would be debating whether ECT works. I hoped that irony wouldn't be lost on the members of the panel. Surely, Andy and I told each other, surely they couldn't look at those bloody pictures, then hear about Jonah's aggression, Matthew's detached retinas, and Paul's catatonic episodes, and vote to restrict the only treatment that ever helped them.

And Jonah isn't alone. There is a growing group of patients whose quality of life depends exclusively on their access to ECT—developmentally delayed kids and teens who suffer from aggressive, self-injurious and catatonic behaviors. I met several of these families over the past year—including a fourteen-year-old autistic boy who was so self-injurious he detached his own retinas—twice! As well as a sixteen-year-old—born with half a cerebellum due to an in-utero stroke—who vacillated between periods of uncontrollable rage and catatonic stupor, during which he would remain frozen, unable to eat, toilet, or communicate, for up to eight days at a time. ECT resolved the extreme behaviors of both these boys, as well as those in other cases reported in the psychiatric literature by doctors at Kennedy Krieger and the University of Michigan, among other places—in fact, Jonah's case was just published in the European Journal of Child and Adolescent Psychiatry.

Behind me, the two-hundred or so seats reserved for spectators were more than half empty. The East Coast had been hit with another snowstorm the day before, stranding many of the interested parties, including witnesses and even members of the panel, several of whom were participating via conference call. Although I had timed my departure to coincide with a break in the blizzard, it had still taken me more than eight hours to make a drive that shouldn't even have taken three, the last four of those hours spent inching along the final twelve miles.

But as agonizing as that ride had been, I appreciated now the storm's effect on the meeting. Notably absent was one of the anti-ECT movement's biggest stars, Leonard Roy Frank, whose testimony was read into the record by an associate, as well as all but a handful of the protestors I had assumed would transform the hearing into a circus. Of course, ECT proponents hadn't been spared either—Kitty Dukakis, scheduled to present to the panel her own life-saving experience with ECT, was so delayed she missed the entire morning session, although I heard the panel agreed to allow her to speak later that afternoon. All in all, I was glad for the relatively calm tenor of the proceedings, which I felt could only help our side.

You will probably hear a lot of people get up and say that ECT doesn't have any long-term benefit. That's because ECT is like dialysis—a treatment, not a cure. Jonah and his terribly afflicted peers need maintenance ECT to keep their symptoms at bay. Which is why I drove eight hours through blinding snow to be here, to implore you to reclassify ECT machines as Class II medical devices, and not to make any decisions that might make ECT less accessible for these children, who need it so desperately.

What will happen if they can't get ECT? Well, the boy who detached his retinas would surely blind himself; the catatonic teen would end up on a feeding tube; and Jonah—Jonah would end up physically or chemically restrained on a locked ward. Instead of where he is now: home, in school, out in the community—enjoying, just like my four other children [and here I held up a blown-up version of our holiday card photo, featuring all five kids on our boat], *a rich, happy, exciting life. Thank you.*

As much as I wanted to stay and watch the rest of the meeting, I left when the panel broke for lunch, allowing plenty of time to get back to Philadelphia for our flight. I felt pretty optimistic about our chances. The panel was made up almost entirely of doctors, a profession I had always trusted for its rationality, intelligence, and genuine desire to help people. It was hard to imagine how these medical professionals could overlook the dozens of studies supporting the safety and efficacy of ECT I knew had been included in the Executive Summary the FDA had prepared for the meeting. And I thought the witnesses who testified in support of ECT were, in general, more credible than those who opposed it. Although two doctors did speak in opposition to reclassification, both are public proponents of non-medical interventions such as "empowerment" and "transformation"—which may in fact help many people, but would be laughably inadequate, not only for Jonah, but also for the bulk of ECT patients, who are typically suicidal, psychotic, catatonic, or manic (and have already failed trials of both psychotherapy and medication). Seven doctors, a nurse, and a nurse practitioner, on the other hand, testified in favor of reclassification. These supporters not only have extensive experience treating the acute patients that desperately need ECT but are actively involved in the most recent ECT research, with academic appointments that include Duke and NYU. Especially compelling was Dr. David Boger, a New York city psychiatrist who also gets regular ECT to control his own incapacitating depression, and who described how he taught a seminar on ECT at Mount Sinai the afternoon after one of his treatments, using himself as Exhibit A to show the absence of side effects.

Several psychiatric patients representing both sides of the debate came, some from great distances, to tell the panel about their experiences with ECT. Perplexingly, two self-designated "psychiatric survivors" had never actually been treated with ECT, although this didn't stop them from condemning it with enormous enthusiasm. I had a great deal of sympathy for other witnesses who reported extensive memory loss, especially for a former Ironman competitor who had packed all her trophies away because she couldn't remember winning them. But of the six who had actually experienced ECT, five had been given their treatments decades ago: thirty, forty, even fifty years ago, before the technological advances that have so drastically reduced these kinds of impairments.

I couldn't help thinking the last witness, although he spoke against ECT, actually supported the other side in his rambling, incoherent account of how he was committed to a psychiatric hospital by his sergeant for violent behavior that he realizes now was caused by . . . a lack of coffee. The rest of this older gentleman's five-minute speech covered everything from the suicide rate in South Korea to a neighbor child his mother had cared for during a long-ago summer, because its mother "had been raised in daycare and she couldn't bond to her baby." I'm not sure what the panel took from that presentation, but I know it reinforced for me the insidious grip of mental illness, the loss of reason and self-awareness, the hopelessness and disconnection—and the sad reality that some of the strongest critics of powerful interventions like ECT and antipsychotics are the people who need them the most. Or I should say, are the people who have benefitted from them the most, because the woman who received her ECT after a suicide attempt is still alive, and the quavering old man who blamed his psychotic episode on a caffeine deficit went on to become, for some part of his life, a physics teacher.

———

Our flight to Orlando was surprisingly, happily, perfectly uneventful. Even though it was so delayed due to the previous day's storm that we didn't reach our rental home until one thirty in the morning, Jonah didn't have one meltdown. We spent our first day at the Magic Kingdom, where Gretchen finally got to meet all the princesses she loved so much (and couldn't actually speak to, she was so overwhelmed). Jonah was very tolerant of all the babyish rides we dragged him on so we could use his handicapped pass and avoid waiting on line. Of course, we also took him on Space Mountain and . . . well, actually Space Mountain was the only ride in the Magic Kingdom that even came close to the thrill of his favorite roller coasters at Six Flags and the amusement piers at the New Jersey shore. I was glad for the twins to experience the magic of Disney, but as we hiked around the park, I decided that I was in no hurry to return. Maybe next winter we would try one of those all-inclusive resorts in the Caribbean. Now that we knew Jonah could travel, we had so many options.

After we left the Magic Kingdom, we stopped for dinner at Outback. While we waited for our table, I emailed Dr. Kellner, who had also been at the meeting and who had planned to stay for the second day. *Just wondering how the deliberations went today*, I wrote, *and whether you had any thoughts about what the panel might recommend to the FDA.*

Badly, replied Dr. Kellner almost immediately. *I'll call you.*

I stared at the tiny letters on my iPhone, exhaling all my buoyancy and good feeling in one long breath. *How could this have happened?* I wondered. *Had these doctors listened, had they read, had they considered . . . ?* I was still staring when the phone vibrated in my hand.

I fumbled my way outside, leaving Andy and Marina to shepherd the kids to our table. Still, the spillover from the restaurant was so great I had to plug my finger into my other ear. "What happened?" I asked.

Dr. Kellner explained that seemingly everything had gone great. After I left, different doctors associated with the FDA had presented meta-analyses confirming the safety and efficacy of ECT. The entire next day had been set aside for deliberations—until, hours early, the Chair of the panel had stopped the debate to take a vote, even though he had announced previously that because their only task was to make general recommendations to the FDA, there would be no vote that day. When the panel split evenly on the issue of whether to reclassify ECT machines to Class II specifically for the indication of major depression, the Chair cast the deciding vote against.

"But they're doctors . . . ," I stammered.

"There were a lot of neurologists on the panel," Dr. Kellner said, including the Chair, as it turned out. "Neurologists as a group have historically opposed ECT. They spend their entire careers trying to stop seizures. They have a tough time understanding how a seizure can be therapeutic."

Later, I would read the transcript of the meeting. I would see how every neurologist and neuropsychologist had, in fact, voted against reclassification for depression, schizophrenia, and bipolar disorder, even while one of them acknowledged, "We all agree it's effective. The data is that it's effective." Every psychiatrist, on the other hand—and these were the only members with first-hand ECT experience—voted in favor; one reminded his colleagues, "There is no equivalent, there is no alternative to ECT for the kinds of patients for which it's used. . . . It is literally lifesaving, and so to eliminate this option would be literally eliminating a lifeline to many patients." I would read how those who most opposed reclassification assured their fellow panelists multiple times that this action "should not have a deleterious effect on the access to ECT"—a claim I found disingenuous since, when pressed by one of the psychiatrists, the Chair admitted that ECT devices would in fact be taken off the market if the manufacturers were unable to design or afford clinical trials of whatever size and scope might be specified by the FDA in its official ruling, which is expected later this year.

Later, I would also learn that the panel had voted to reclassify for one indication—catatonia—and this would give me hope that ECT for the young people in this book would never be disrupted. Not only do many of them already have a diagnosis of catatonia, but virtually all the rest exhibit some catatonic symptoms, including purposeless, agitated motor activity (such as pounding one's self in the face hundreds of times); stereotyped movement; echolalia (repeating another's speech); and negativism (resistance to all directions).

But at that moment, first hearing the news in front of the Outback, I was speechless, trying to process what I was hearing.

"The good news is that the government moves glacially," Dr. Kellner continued. "We shouldn't see any further restrictions for three or four years."

"Great," I said faintly. Since neither Dr. Kellner nor I were doing a terribly good job bucking each other up, we said our goodbyes.

"Thanks again for testifying," he said in closing. "Yours was the best speech of the meeting."

"Thanks," I said. I clicked off my phone, thinking, *Not good enough.*

I pushed my way back into the Outback, wondering—as I had several times over the past year—if there was any chance at all that I could be the crazy one. Because if it's not me, then it's all of them.

The neurologists. The Scientologists. The thousands of members of anti-psychiatry groups in general and anti-ECT organizations in particular that lobby for the abolition of ECT. The 61 percent of voters in Berkeley, California who voted to ban ECT within the city limits in 1982. If it's not me, then all of them must be—not crazy, necessarily, but absolutely wrong. And it's hard to wrap your mind around the possibility that so many people could be so aggressively, fervently, immovably wrong, especially when it's not about a metaphysical issue like the existence of God but about such a seemingly simple and answerable question like whether or not ECT helps people.

Halfway across the room I could see my family seated at a round table. The kids were scribbling on their children's menus, Andy was picking at a Bloomin' Onion, and Jonah was waiting patiently for the "ketchup and one THOUSAND hamburgers and French fries" he had ordered. And I knew, with absolute certainty, that I wasn't crazy. I saw in my mind everything we had done that day: Jonah trailing his fingers through the Small World canal; leaning on me while the other kids watched the princes and princesses sing and dance in front of Cinderella's castle; walking without complaint the endless miles we logged crossing and re-crossing the Magic Kingdom. And then I saw Jonah at home: breezing through a multiplication worksheet, horsing around with Andy during his swimming lesson, climbing to the very top of the rock wall gym. How ridiculous to doubt, when Jonah's transformation was nothing short of miraculous. As difficult as it was to accept that so many people could be wrong, I lived with the proof of it every day.

I took my seat next to Jonah, signaling in response to Andy's questioning look that we would talk later, once the kids were asleep. But even as I buttered a piece of bread for Aaron and admired the amazingly lifelike rendition of a palomino horse Erika had somehow drawn with only two dulled crayons, I knew we had no choice but to do what we have always taught our kids to do when the world throws obstacles in our paths: keep fighting.

Afterword, May 16, 2013

What comes after epilogue: *postscript, coda, addendum?* Because Jonah's story is of course ongoing, and will continue on—I hope for many, many years.

As this book goes to press, Jonah is fourteen years old. He has been receiving ECT for just over three years and has gotten approximately 136 treatments. His behavior is still, overall, phenomenally stable, but he hasn't gone through puberty yet, so that particular question is yet to be answered. Although there have been blips in his level of agitation, we have seen no aggression at all at home. He has hit his teacher a couple of times, but nothing like the attacks he was capable of in the pre-ECT days, when he would scramble over desks and chairs to launch himself at his target with unfettered ferocity. In fact, next month he is transferring schools: the first time in his life that he is moving to a less, not more, restrictive environment. Jonah will be attending the Preparing Adolescents and Adults for Life (PAAL) Program, an amazing secondary school for students with moderate to severe autism that does virtually all its teaching out in the community. Students shop in local stores; cook, clean and do laundry in homes owned by the school; exercise in a neighborhood gym; and work at jobs with various community partners, including restaurants and offices. There are excursions to Broadway shows, summer vacations at the Jersey shore, and trips to an extreme sports camp in Colorado. But what excites me the most is a video on the PAAL website (*www.mecaautism.org/paal.html*) in which an autistic teenager walks into a convenience store all by himself, wearing a Bluetooth earpiece. He picks out his items, waits in line, and checks out while his teacher watches through the storefront window, prompting him over the phone: "Say 'credit' . . . Good job!" It's almost impossible for me to imagine Jonah going into a convenience store by himself without grabbing bags of chips or candy, ripping them apart, and shoving as much as he can into his mouth before he's caught. But the director of PAAL says that Jonah will be able to do exactly that. As heartbreaking as it will be for both Jonah and me to say goodbye to the incredibly supportive staff at Milagre, I can't wait to see what else he will learn to do in the world.

Keri, Matty, and their kids moved out in March 2011. They bought a house about five minutes away. Our kids go to the same schools and we see them frequently, but there's definitely been an atmospheric shift. As I noted to Marina shortly after they left, knowing as I said it how crazy it would sound to most people, "It's so quiet around here with only five kids in the house."

Jonah gets ECT every nine or ten days, depending on how the weekend falls. We did try to extend the time between treatments to eleven or twelve days about a year and a half ago, but after three cycles, he ended up punching out a window, so we dropped back down. Thankfully, there have been no legal threats to Jonah's maintenance ECT. As worried as I was about potential action by the FDA, there has been no response by that organization to the recommendations of the advisory panel more than two years ago. ECT machines remain in the same limbo they have been in for decades—which is a relief, because we can't afford to lose any weapons in the fight to treat dangerous behaviors in the developmentally disabled. This has turned out to be an even bigger problem than was previously thought. While earlier research estimated that up to a third of autistic individuals suffer from aggressive and/or self-injurious behaviors, a 2013 study out of the University of Missouri-Columbia reported aggression in over *half* of autistic kids aged two to seventeen.[1] This retrospective study was unable to determine the severity of the aggression or its responsiveness to different therapies. But it's impossible not to see this staggering figure as a mandate for more awareness, more research, and more effective treatments for this problem in this population.

The role ECT will play in this schema remains uncertain. Research continues to pour in from all over the world. PubMed cites more than eight hundred new ECT studies published since January 2011. About twenty focus on young patients, including a 2012 Chinese study that randomly assigned adolescent, psychotic patients into two groups, one of which was given psychotropic medication while the other received ECT in conjunction with medication. Researchers found the patients in the ECT group had shorter hospital stays and showed greater improvement than those who were treated with medication alone.[2] Case reports document the successful treatment of adolescents using ECT in India, France, Germany, and the Czech Republic,[3] as well as at respected American institutions such as Washington University, University of Michigan, Ohio State University, Spring Harbor Hospital in Maine, and even KKI, the sponsoring institution on Jonah's case study, which became part of the official psychiatric literature when it was published in *European Journal of Child and Adolescent Psychiatry* in 2011.[4] And researchers continue to test young patients for any cognitive impairments post-ECT. One Spanish study compared two groups of schizophrenic adolescents, only one of which was treated with ECT. Investigators found that a neuropsychological battery two years later revealed no differences between the groups.

But the fact remains that no researcher will be able to produce the type of experiment skeptics clamor for and government agencies require: the randomized, controlled, double-blind study, which randomly divides similarly afflicted patients at similar developmental levels into two groups, one of which is given ECT while the other receives the same general anesthesia and muscle relaxants, but no electrical stimulus and no seizure.

It's not impossible to execute such experiments; "sham ECT" has been compared to the real deal in a dozen studies dating back to 1956. But the population of autistic kids with dangerous behaviors raises unique challenges to such a study. First of all, these kids have such complicated histories that it would be difficult to match them to one another, which is necessary to isolate the variable being tested— namely, the efficacy of ECT. But an even greater obstacle is the ethics of taking kids as severely afflicted as Jonah, Matthew, Paul, Gary, and David were—patients at risk every day of seriously hurting themselves or others—and giving them a placebo. Who would be liable if Matthew blinded himself, or Jonah bludgeoned his youngest sister? What parent, what researcher, what hospital or university administrators would take that risk?

Interestingly, we inadvertently performed such an experiment earlier this year. One treatment cycle in March, Jonah had much higher levels of agitation than we had seen in many months. He bloodied his own nose repeatedly, grabbed at his teacher, and lost all interest in his most preferred activities. He was constantly unhappy and struggling (but often failing) to keep his composure. Dr. Wachtel and I exchanged emails over whether Jonah's medications needed adjustment; I took him in for a blood test to check his lithium level. While we were waiting for the results, Marina took him in for his next scheduled ECT. When the doctor found out how terrible Jonah's week had been, he told Marina that he wasn't surprised: Jonah's seizure the previous session had only lasted sixteen seconds. Seizures under thirty seconds don't elicit the physiological changes caused by ECT and aren't considered therapeutic.

Thankfully, we haven't had to worry about Jonah's behavior since, because now that I don't have to spend the bulk of my time managing my son's tantrums I've been busy with other activities. In 2011 I started—with Michael Dinda and Mike Eisert, another father of an autistic teen—EASI Foundation: Ending Aggression and Self-Injury in the Developmentally Disabled. This isn't an ECT advocacy group, but a support for families of individuals with autism and dangerous behaviors. Our first project was to construct a nationwide resource guide of child psychiatrists, schools, camps, equipment vendors, and ECT providers that service this population. As Lisa, Alex's mom, observed, "You're at the mercy of whoever you can find to work with." We just want to spare other parents the incredibly circuitous, frustrating journeys we all took with our kids, and connect them with help, in whatever form they need it, as quickly as possible.

Acknowledgments

If it takes a village to raise a typical child, it takes a city to raise one as challenging as Jonah was before his mood was stabilized with ECT. I am so grateful to the incredible support system that got us through those desperate years:

Keri and Matty—I honestly don't know how I would have made it through the time period covered in this book without you. I could fill another volume with all the things you've done for us, but I'll choose one: thank you for embracing Jonah, for not being afraid of him, even on behalf of your own children. This wasn't your problem, yet you made it your problem, and I will be forever grateful for that.

Marina and Oat—I don't think you could love my kids any more if they were your own. You have really become part of our family, and that has given me tremendous peace of mind. Marina, I bet when you signed on as our nanny you never thought you would end up as an experienced therapeutic staff support (TSS), but you couldn't run Jonah's behavior plan any better if you had a string of letters after your name.

Lauren—is there anything you can't do? Thanks for being my favorite author-photo photographer, Apple goddess, and reliable coffee klatcher.

We've been fortunate to have an amazing home team. It's impossible for me to remember everyone who has worked with Jonah since he was five, as the team frequently evolved, and I apologize for leaving anyone out. Thanks Melissa Sterner, Shannon Herbert, Cheri Settanni, Rael Lapenta, Emily Dillon, Jennifer Nelson, Lauren Scott, Chelsea Andrews, Candace Williams, Isabel Tinker, Joaquin Galarza, Keryn Koch, Zach Groff, Nick Taugner, Ashley Bockman, Lauren Naile, Amanda Mason, Maria Kioukis, Theresa Everett, and Heather Paul. I have told anyone who would listen that those who choose to work with this very difficult population are simply the finest human beings out there, and I'm grateful for the opportunity to know all of you.

Thanks to everyone at the Milagre Kids School for their patience, perseverance, and for never making us feel that Jonah wasn't welcome, no matter how badly his behavior deteriorated. Thanks especially to the beloved Mr. Boss, Tricia Cuce, Sharon Keppley, Trish Fisher, Melissa Lambert, and Nicole Davis.

Jonah has had caring, dedicated doctors to guide us along his entire journey, including Jeff Bomze, James Hetznecker, and Richard Jaffe and the entire staff at Belmont Behavioral Health. But I have to single out two unbelievable doctors who changed our lives forever: Lee Wachtel and Charles Kellner. Thank you so, so much for giving us our son back. Your commitment to him and to the population of kids with developmental delay and dangerous behaviors is awe-inspiring.

Bringing this story to publication took three long years, and I have to thank my champions: Susan Ramer, my unbelievably dedicated agent, and Michael Ames, my editor at Vanderbilt University Press, who believed in this manuscript from the first time he saw it and never gave up on it. Thanks also to Charles Kellner (again) and Dirk Dhossche for their insightful foreword, and even more for supporting this project enough to attach their names to it.

Thanks so much to the families that shared their stories with me. Your suffering has shattered me, your ferocity has humbled me, and your strength has inspired me.

Finally, my own fabulous family. Jonah, Erika, Hilary, Aaron, and Gretchen, it is a privilege to parent each and every one of you. You enrich my life in countless ways every day and I love you MOST. Andy—I can't imagine a better partner for this journey, which has been so very different from what we imagined when we set out together sixteen years ago. Throughout it all you have been a wonderful husband and an even better father. You are the Jonah Whisperer.

Notes

CHAPTER 1

1. Kitty Dukakis and Larry Tye, *Shock: The Healing Power of Electroconvulsive Therapy* (New York: Penguin Group, 2006).

2. J. W. Thompson and J. D. Blaine, "Use of ECT in the United States in 1975 and 1980," *American Journal of Psychiatry* 144 (1987): 557–62.

3. N. Ghaziuddin, D. Laughrin, and B. Giordani, "Cognitive Side Effects of Electroconvulsive Therapy in Adolescents," *Journal of Child and Adolescent Psychopharmacology* 10 (2000): 269–76.

4. Sandra G. Boodman, "Shock Therapy . . . It's Back," *Washington Post*, September 24, 1996.

5. Treatments "work" when they cause a remission of psychiatric symptoms as assessed with various testing instruments. For example, in determining whether an antidepressant treatment (like Prozac or ECT) works, a researcher would compare scores on assessments like the Hamilton Rating Scale for Depression (HSRD) pre- and post-treatment. But mood psychiatric disorders are chronic, episodic conditions, and there is no permanent medical cure. More generally, a treatment "works" when it improves a patient's ability to function, which has always been the goal of psychiatric interventions.

6. Lauretta Bender, "One Hundred Cases of Childhood Schizophrenia Treated with Electric Shock," *Transactions of the American Neurological Association* 72 (1947): 165–69.

7. E. R. Clardy and Elizabeth M. Rumpf, "The Effect of Electric Shock Treatment on Children Having Schizophrenic Manifestations," *Psychiatric Quarterly* 4 (1954): 616–23.

8. J. M. Rey and G. Walter, "Half a Century of ECT Use in Young People," *American Journal of Psychiatry* 154 (1997): 595–602.

9. See D. Cohen et al., "Absence of Cognitive Impairment at Long-Term Follow-Up in Adolescents Treated with ECT for Severe Mood Disorder," *American Journal of Psychiatry* 157 (2000): 460–62; and O. Taieb et al., "Clinical Relevance of Electroconvulsive Therapy (ECT) in Adolescents with Severe Mood Disorder: Evidence from a Follow-Up Study," *European Psychiatry* 17 (2002): 206–12.

10. Ghaziuddin, Laughrin, and Giordani, "Cognitive Side Effects," 273.

11. S. Kazumasa et al., "Improvement of Psychiatric Symptoms after Electroconvulsive Therapy in Young Adults with Intractable First-Episode Schizo-

phrenia and Schizophreniform Disorder," *Journal of Experimental Medicine* 210 (2006): 213–20.

12. M. Fink, "Complaints of Loss of Personal Memories after Electroconvulsive Therapy: Evidence of a Somatoform Disorder?" *Psychosomatics* 48 (2007): 290–93.

13. National Institutes of Health Consensus Development Conference Statement: Electroconvulsive Therapy. June 10–12, 1985, *consensus.nih.gov/1985/1985electroconvulsivetherapy051html.htm*.

14. H. Sackeim et al., "The Cognitive Effects of Electroconvulsive Therapy in Community Settings," *Neuropsychopharmacology* 32 (2007): 244–54.

15. American Psychiatric Association, Committee on Electroconvulsive Therapy, Richard D. Weiner (chairperson) et al., *The Practice of Electroconvulsive Therapy: Recommendations For Treatment, Training, and Privileging (2nd ed.)* (Washington, DC: American Psychiatric Publishing, 2001).

16. M. F. Newman et al., "Longitudinal Assessment of Neurocognitive Function after Coronary-Artery Bypass Surgery," *New England Journal of Medicine* 344 (2001): 395–402.

CHAPTER 3

1. Quoted in Edward Shorter and David Healy, *Shock Therapy: A History of Electroconvulsive Treatment in Mental Illness* (New Brunswick: Rutgers University Press, 2007), 2.

2. Frank's letter is available at *goo.gl/17isGv*.

3. C. Kellner et al. "Continuation Electroconvulsive Therapy vs. Pharmacotherapy for Relapse Prevention in Major Depression," *Archives of General Psychiatry* 63 (2006): 1337–44.

4. M. Trivedi et al., "Evaluation of Outcomes with Citalopram for Depression Using Measurement-Based Care in STAR*D: Implications for Clinical Practice," *American Journal of Psychiatry* 163 (2006): 28–40.

5. C. Kellner et al., "Relief of Expressed Suicidal Intent by ECT: A Consortium for Research in ECT Study," *American Journal of Psychiatry* 162 (2005): 977–82.

6. M. Gliatto et al., "Evaluation and Treatment of Patients with Suicidal Ideation," *American Family Physician Bulletin*, March 15, 1999.

7. See S. Brandon et al., "Electroconvulsive Therapy: Results in Depressive Illness from the Leicestershire Trial," *British Medical Journal* 288 (1984): 22–25; and S. Mukherjee and H. A. Sackeim, "Electroconvulsive Therapy of Acute Manic Episodes: A Review of 50 Years' Experience," *American Journal of Psychiatry* 151 (1994): 169–76.

8. See L. Wachtel et al., "Electroconvulsive Therapy in a Man with Autism Experiencing Severe Depression, Catatonia, and Self Injury," *Journal of ECT* 26 (2010): 70–73; and J. N. Trollor and P. A. Sachdev, "Electroconvulsive Treat-

ment of Neuroleptic Malignant Syndrome: A Review and Report of Cases," *Australian and New Zealand Journal of Psychiatry* 33 (1999): 650–59.

9. J. Rey and G. Walter, "Half a Century of ECT Use in Young People," *American Journal of Psychiatry* 154 (1997): 595–602.

10. S. Kutcher and H. Robertson, "Electroconvulsive Therapy in Treatment-Resistant Bipolar Youth," *Journal of Child and Adolescent Psychopharmacology* 5 (1995): 167–75.

11. N. Ghaziuddin et al., "Electroconvulsive Treatment in Adolescents with Pharmachotherapy-Refractory Depression," *Journal of Child and Adolescent Psychopharmacology* 6 (1996): 259–71.

12. M. Strober, "Effects of Electroconvulsive Therapy in Adolescents with Severe Endogenous Depression Resistant to Pharmacotherapy," *Biological Psychiatry* 43 (1998): 335–38.

13. J. D. Little et al., "ECT Use Delayed in the Presence of Comorbid Mental Retardation: A Review of Clinical and Ethical Issues," *The Journal of ECT* 18 (2002): 218–22.

14. Linda Andre, *Doctors of Deception: What They Don't Want You to Know about Shock Treatment* (New Brunswick: Rutgers University Press, 2009), 271.

15. Peter Breggin, *Brain-Disabling Treatments in Psychiatry: Drugs, Electroshock, and the Psychopharmaceutical Complex* (New York: Springer Publishing Company, 2008), 226.

16. C. Ross, "The Sham ECT Literature: Implications for Consent to ECT," *Ethical Human Psychology and Psychiatry* 8 (2006): 17–28.

17. University of Louisville School of Medicine, "1,250 Electroconvulsive Treatments without Evidence of Brain Injury" *British Journal of Psychiatry* 147 (1985): 203–4.

18. D. P. Devanand et al., "Absence of Cognitive Impairment After More Than 100 Lifetime ECT Treatments," *American Journal of Psychiatry* 148 (1991): 929–32.

CHAPTER 5

1. C. P. L. Freeman and R. E. Kendell, "ECT: I. Patients' Experiences and Attitudes," *British Journal of Psychiatry* 137 (1980): 8–16.

CHAPTER 6

1. Lorna Wing and Amitta Shah, "Catatonia in Autistic Spectrum Disorders," *British Journal of Psychiatry* 29 (2000): 357–62.

2. US Department of Health and Human Services, *Mental Health: A Report of the Surgeon General*, (Rockville, MD: US Department of Health and Human Services, Substance Abuse and Mental Health Services Administration, Center for Mental Health Services, National Institutes of Health, National Institute of Mental Health, 1999).

CHAPTER 8

1. C. Kellner et al., "Bifrontal, Bitemporal and Right Unilateral Electrode Placement in ECT: Randomized Trial," *The British Journal of Psychiatry* 196 (2010): 226–34.

CHAPTER 9

1. Kutcher and Robertson, "Electroconvulsive Therapy," 171.

2. Judith Warner, *We've Got Issues: Children and Parents in the Age of Medication* (New York: Riverhead Books, 2010), 3.

CHAPTER 11

1. Charles Kellner, *Brain Stimulation in Psychiatry: ECT, DBS, TMS and Other Modalities* (Cambridge: Cambridge University Press, 2012), 7.

2. M. Fink, "Neuroendocrine Predictors of Electroconvulsive Therapy Outcome. Dexamethasone Suppression Test and Prolactin," *Annals of the New York Academy of Sciences* 462 (1986): 30–36.

3. C. M. Marano et al., "Increased Plasma Concentration of Brain-Derived Neurotrophic Factor with Electroconvulsive Therapy: A Pilot Study in Patients with Major Depression. *Journal of Clinical Psychiatry* 68 (2007): 512–17.

4. B. W. Scott et al., "Neurogenesis in the Dentate Gyrus of the Rat Following Electroconvulsive Shock Seizures," *Experimental Neurology* 165, no. 2 (October 2000): 231–36.

5. F. Chen et al., "Repeated Electroconvulsive Seizures Increase the Total Number of Synapses in Adult Male Rat Hippocampus," *European Neuropsychopharmacology* 19, no. 5 (2009): 329–38.

6. Henrietta van Praag, Barry Jacobs, and Fred Gage, "Depression and the Birth and Death of Brain Cells," *American Scientist* 88 (July–August 2000): 340–45.

7. P. Nordanskog et al., "Increase in Hippocampal Volume After Electroconvulsive Therapy in Patients with Depression: A Volumetric Magnetic Resonance Imaging Study," *Journal of ECT* 26, no. 1, (2010): 62–67.

8. M. S. Nobler et al., "Decreased Regional Brain Metabolism After ECT," *American Journal of Psychiatry* 158 (2001): 305–8.

9. J. S. Perrin et al., "Electroconvulsive Therapy Reduces Frontal Cortical Connectivity in Severe Depressive Disorder," *Proceedings of the National Academy of Sciences USA* 109 (2012): 5464–68.

10. S. H. Lisanby et al., "Safety and Feasibility of Magnetic Seizure Therapy (MST) in Major Depression: Randomized Within-Subject Comparison with Electroconvulsive Therapy," *Neuropsychopharmacology* 28 (2003): 1852–65.

11. Peter R. Breggin, *Toxic Psychiatry: Why Therapy, Empathy and Love Must Replace the Drugs, Electroshock, and Biochemical Theories of the "New Psychiatry"* (New York: St. Martin's Press, 1991), 198.

1. This calculation assumes a 350 million steady-state population multiplied by the estimated autism rate of .67 percent, multiplied by the aggressive/SIB rate of .28, which equals 650,000 instances.

2. G. H. Murphy et al., "Chronicity of Challenging Behaviours in People with Severe Intellectual Disabilities and/or Autism: A Total Population Sample," *Journal of Autism and Developmental Disorders* 35 (2005): 405–18.

3. Thomas Szasz, *The Myth of Mental Illness: Foundations of a Theory of Personal Conduct* (New York: HarperCollins, 1960), 182.

4. Szasz, *The Myth of Mental Illness*, 259.

5. "Testimony of Leonard Roy Frank at a public hearing on electroconvulsive 'treatment' before the Mental Health Committee of the New York State Assembly, Martin A. Luster (chairman), Manhattan, 18 May 2001," available at *www.ect.org/news/newyork/franktest.html.*

6. Breggin, *Toxic Psychiatry*, 290.

7. David Eagleman, *Incognito: The Secret Lives of the Brain* (New York: Pantheon Books, 2011), 172.

8. See R. E. Rosenberg et al., "Characteristics and Concordance of Autism Spectrum Disorders Among 277 Twin Pairs," *Archives of Pediatric and Adolescent Medicine* 163 (2009): 907–14; J. Lau, and T. Eley, "The Genetics of Mood Disorders," *Annual Review of Clinical Psychology* 6 (2010): 313–37; A. C. Van der Schot et al., "Genetic and Environmental Influences on Focal Brain Density in Bipolar Disorder," *Brain* 133 (2010): 3080–89; and R. A. Shih et al., "A Review of the Evidence from Family, Twin and Adoption Studies for a Genetic Contribution to Adult Psychiatric Disorders," *International Review of Psychiatry* 16 (2004): 260–83.

9. D. Dhossche and U. Rout, "Are Autistic and Catatonic Regression Related? A Few Working Hypotheses Involving GABA, Purkinje Cell Survival, Neurogenesis, and ECT," *International Review of Neurobiology* 72 (2006): 55–79.

10. See D. E. Arking et al., "A Common Genetic Variant in the Neurexin Superfamily Member CNTNAP2 Increases Familial Risk of Autism," *American Journal of Human Genetics* 82 (2008): 160–64; L. A. Weiss et al., "Association Between Microdeletion and Microduplication at 16p11.2 and Autism," *New England Journal of Medicine* 358 (2008): 667–75; and S. Jamain et al., "Mutations of the XLinked Genes Encoding Neuroligins NLGN3 and NLGN4 Are Associated with Autism," *Nature Genetics* 34 (2003): 27–29

11. See C. A. Matthews, and V. I. Reus, "Genetic Linkage in Bipolar Disorder," *CNS Spectrums* 8 (2003): 891–904; and V. Abkevich et al., "Predisposition Locus for Major Depression at Chromosome 12q22–12q23.2," *The American Journal of Human Genetics* 73 (2003): 1271–81.

12. D. Weinberger, "Biological Phenotypes and Genetic Research on Schizophrenia," *World Psychiatry* 1 (February 2002): 2–6.

13. Breggin, *Toxic Psychiatry*, 374.

14. Andre, *Doctors of Deception*, 2.

15. L. Frank, "Psychiatry's Unholy Trinity—Fraud, Fear and Force: A Personal Account," *Ideas on Liberty*, November 2002: 23–27.

AFTERWORD

1. M. O. Mazurek, S. M. Kanne, and E. L. Wodka, "Physical Aggression in Children and Adolescents with Autism Spectrum Disorders," *Research in Autism Spectrum Disorders* 7 (2013): 455–65.

2. Zhang-Jin Zhang et al., "Electroconvulsive Therapy Improves Antipsychotic and Somnographic Responses in Adolescents with First-Episode Psychosis—A Case-Control Study," *Schizophrenia Research* 137 (2012): 97–103.

3. See S. Grover et al., "Electroconvulsive Therapy in Adolescents: A Retrospective Study from North India," *Journal of ECT* (2013) [Electronic preprint]; A. Consoli et al., "Electroconvulsive Therapy in Adolescents with Intellectual Disability and Severe Self-Injurious Behavior and Aggression: A Retrospective Study," *European Journal of Child and Adolescent Psychiatry* 22 (2013): 55–62; F. Habler et al, "A Case of Catatonia in a 14-Year-Old Girl with Schizophrenia Treated with Electroconvulsive Therapy," *Zeitschrift fur Kinder-und Jugendpsychiatrie und Psychotherapie* 41 (2013): 69–74; and M. Goetz et al., "Combined Use of Electroconvulsive Therapy and Amantadine in Adolescent Catatonia Precipitated by Cyber-Bullying," *Journal of Child and Adolescent Psychopharmacology* 23 (2013): 228–31.

4. See T. Mon et al., "The Use Of Electroconvulsive Therapy in a Patient with Juvenile Systemic Lupus Erythematosus and Catatonia," *Lupus* 21 (2012): 1575–81; S. N. Jap and N. Ghaziuddin, "Catatonia Among Adolescents with Down Syndrome: A Review and 2 Case Reports," *Journal of ECT* 27 (2011): 334–37; J. C. Rhoads et al, "The Successful Use of Right Unilateral Ultra-Brief Pulse Electroconvulsive Therapy in an Adolescent with Catatonia," *Brain Stimulation* 3 (2010):51–53; M. Siegel et al., "Electroconvulsive Therapy in an Adolescent with Autism and Bipolar I Disorder," *Journal of ECT* 28 (2012): 252–55; and L. E. Wachtel et al., "Electroconvulsive Therapy for Psychotropic-Refractory Bipolar Affective Disorder and Severe Self-Injury and Aggression in an 11-Year-Old Autistic Boy," *European Journal of Child and Adolescent Psychiatry* 20 (2011): 147–52.

Index

Aberrant Behavior Checklist (ABC), 94
Abilify, 3, 38–39, 130, 176
aggression
    in Alex, 126–28
    in Jonah, 1–4, 7, 40, 42, 81–83, 90,
        139–41, 175
    in Matthew, 26–27
    in Paul, 46–49, 56
    prevalence rates in the autistic
        population, 161–62, 186
    prognosis over time, 29, 54
    reduction with ECT, 27, 56, 84, 92,
        178, 185
alternative treatments in autism, 2, 7,
    24, 68–69, 129, 152
American Psychiatric Association
    (APA), 170–71, 177
Andre, Linda, 17–18, 36, 160, 168–69,
    171, 193n14
antipsychotics, 46, 100, 154, 176, 181
    side effects of, 3, 6–7, 24, 34, 54,
        98–99, 130, 135
    See also individual drugs
Apple, Jeff, 172
Autism Diagnostic Observation
    Schedule (ADOS), 93–94

Bailine, Samuel, 73–74
Bauer, Ann, 69
behavior plans, 4, 27, 31, 81, 94, 119,
    137, 146
Behrman, Andy, 172
Belmont Center for Comprehensive
    Care, 93, 123–27, 133–34, 190
Bender, Lauretta, 15, 191n6
benzodiazepines, xiii, xv, 17, 48, 130

bipolar disorder
    in Alex, 130, 133
    genetics of, 165–66
    as an indication for ECT, 38,
        183
    in Jonah, 3, 20, 38, 119
    and maintenance ECT, 141–42
    remission with ECT, xiii
    in Sam, 99–106
Boger, David, 180
Boss, Nick, 55, 62, 83–84, 91, 124–
    125, 190
Breggin, Peter, 36, 147–48, 164–65,
    168, 172, 193n15, 194n11
Brewis, Kathy, 169
Brown, Ian, 113

Camp Joy, 89–90, 120–23
catatonia
    AACAP presentation on, 156
    in autism, xv
    FDA reclassification of ECT for,
        183
    in Gary and David, 71–74
    genetics of, 166
    in Paul, 48–50
    remission with ECT, 34–35, 37, 69,
        74
Cavett, Dick, 172
Chabasinski, Ted, 15
Children's Hospital of Philadelphia
    (CHOP), 9–11
Clozaril, 54, 134, 137
Consortium for Research in ECT
    (CORE), 34, 102, 192n5
Cott, Jonathan, 19

depression
  in David, 72, 74
  genetics of, 165–66
  and maintenance ECT, 141–42
  remission with ECT, xiii, 34–35, 74
Dhossche, Dirk, xi–xv, 156, 195n9
Dukakis, Kitty, 14, 16, 142, 172, 179,
  191n1

Eagleman, David, 165
EASI Foundation: Ending
  Aggression and Self-Injury in the
  Developmentally Disabled, 188
ect.org, 13, 17, 36, 169, 195n5
electroconvulsive therapy (ECT)
  access to, 14, 21, 32–33, 170, 176,
    178–79, 183
  acute course, xiii, 87, 132, 158
  administration of, xiii, 5, 61
  Berkeley ban of, 33, 184
  children and adolescents in, xiii–xiv,
    14–16, 34–35, 186–87
  controversy, xii, 5, 19, 36, 105–6,
    160–73
  cost of, 37, 50, 106, 144
  efficacy, xii–xiii, xv, 14, 34–37,
    186–87
  electrode placement in, 12, 101–2,
    142, 194n1 (chap. 8), 196n4
  FDA regulation of, 170–71, 175–84
  history, xii, 14
  indications, xii–xiii, 182–83
  involuntary, 73–74
  maintenance, xiii, xv, 29, 37, 50–51,
    104, 122, 141–42, 186
  mechanism of action of, xiv, 142–43
  safety of, 61–62
  "sham," 37, 187–88, 193n16
  side effects of, xiv–xv, 15–20, 37–
    38, 50–51, 92, 102–3, 170, 181
  unmodified, xii, 15, 170
  utilization rates, 14, 161

Fink, Max, 17, 33–34, 156, 192n12,
  194n2 (chap. 11)

Fisher, Carrie, 172
Frank, Leonard Roy, 33, 164–65, 169,
  179, 192n2, 195n5, 196n15

genetics of mental illness, 165–66
Ghaziuddin, Neera, 156, 191n3, 196n4

Hetznecker, James, 38, 107

Individuals with Disabilities Education
  Act (IDEA), 41–42

Jaffe, Richard, 93, 117, 123–24, 127,
  133, 158
Johnson, Stewart, 84–85

Kellner, Charles
  AACAP presentation by, 156
  accessibility of, 107, 120
  assessments of Jonah's response
    to ECT, 82, 84, 86–87, 89–90,
    92–93, 123
  criticism of, by anti-ECT groups, 13,
    106
  ECT administration by, 61–64, 76
  and FDA hearing, 182–83
  initial meeting with, 12–14, 16, 20–21
  introduction by, xi–xv
  and Mount Sinai ethics committee,
    32–33, 39, 42–43
  research by, 34, 102, 192n3, 194n1
    (chap. 8), 194n1 (chap. 11)
Kennedy Krieger Institute (KKI), 3–8,
  20, 22–29, 38–41, 119, 144, 187
  See also neurobehavioral unit
Kingsley, Emily Perl, 88
Klein, Donald, 71–73
Kolevzon, Alexander, 52–58, 61, 84–85,
  92–94, 134, 160

lithium, 3, 38–39, 49, 76, 100, 130,
  157, 176

Manning, Martha, ix, 16, 172
memantine, 145–47, 157

Metrazol, 144
Milagre School, 126, 186, 190
Mount Sinai Hospital, xi, 11–14, 60–
   63, 77, 82, 101, 120–24, 155
Mukhopadhyay, Tito, 54–55
Muller, Liz, 52, 62–65, 77, 88–92, 101,
   120

neurobehavioral unit, 13, 21, 94. *See
   also* Kennedy Krieger Institute
neurogenesis, xiv, 142–43, 194n4
neuroleptic malignant syndrome, 6, 34,
   100, 193–94n8
Nuland, Sherwin B., 16–17, 37, 172

PACU (post-anesthesia care unit), 61,
   63, 77, 82, 89–92, 123
Pediatric Autoimmune
   Neuropsychiatric Disorders
   Associated with Streptococcal
   Infections (PANDAS), 129, 154–55
plasmapheresis, 154–55
Plath, Sylvia, 169–70
Popeo, Dennis, 90–91
Preparing Adolescents and Adults for
   Life (PAAL), 185–86
Private Practice, 166–67

residential treatment facilities (RTFs),
   xi, 23, 39–42, 54–56, 134–37, 145,
   152–58
restraint, 7, 25, 27, 47, 61, 134–35,
   141, 162–63
Rey, Joseph, 34–35, 191n8, 193n9
Risperdal, 7, 38, 46–48, 141

One Flew Over the Cuckoo's Nest,
   (Kesey), xi–xii, 5, 154

Sackeim, Harold 17–19, 192n14,
   192n7 (chap. 3)
Salters, Peggy, 17

Scientology, Church of, 5, 163–64,
   171
self-injurious behavior (SIB)
   in Alex, 134
   in John, 157
   in Jonah, 38, 40, 43, 80, 175
   in Matthew, 22–23, 26–27
   prevalence rates in the autistic
      population, 161–62
   prognosis over time, 29, 54
   reduction with ECT, 27, 94, 178–79
Seroussi, Karyn, 7
Shestack, Jonathan, 87–88
Steuernagel, Trudy, 8, 176
suicide, 34
Szasz, Thomas, 163

TSO (tricuris suis ova), 84–85

van Hoom, Ed, 160–61
Versed, 52, 63, 91, 123–24

Wachtel, Lee
   accessibility of, 4, 107
   consultation on Alex, 134
   on interdisciplinary approach to
      treatment, 137
   on maintenance ECT, 121–23, 141
   previous patients treated with ECT,
      4–7, 33, 141
   research and presentations by,
      50–51, 140, 192n8, 196n4
   treatment of John, 155, 157
   treatment of Jonah , 20, 38–39,
      145–46, 149
   treatment of Matthew, 23
   treatment of Paul, 48–51
Walter, Garry, 34–35, 191n8, 193n9
Warner, Judith, 6, 106–7, 194n2
   (chap. 9)
Wilson, Adam, 172
Wynette, Tammy, 172